THE ENDOCRINE SYSTEM

GENERAL EDITORS

Dale C. Garell, M.D.
Medical Director, California Children Services, Department of Health
 Services, County of Los Angeles
Associate Dean for Curriculum
Clinical Professor, Department of Pediatrics & Family Medicine,
 University of Southern California School of Medicine
Former President, Society for Adolescent Medicine

Solomon H. Snyder, M.D.
Distinguished Service Professor of Neuroscience, Pharmacology, and
 Psychiatry, Johns Hopkins University School of Medicine
Former president, Society of Neuroscience
Albert Lasker Award in Medical Research, 1978

CONSULTING EDITORS

Robert W. Blum, M.D., Ph.D.
Associate Professor, School of Public Health and Department of
 Pediatrics
Director, Adolescent Health Program, University of Minnesota
Consultant, World Health Organization

Charles E. Irwin, Jr., M.D.
Associate Professor of Pediatrics; Director, Division of Adolescent
 Medicine, University of California, San Francisco

Lloyd J. Kolbe, Ph.D.
Chief, Office of School Health & Special Projects, Center for Health
 Promotion & Education, Centers for Disease Control
President, American School Health Association

Jordan J. Popkin
Director, Division of Federal Employee Occupational Health, U.S. Public
 Health Service Region I

Joseph L. Rauh, M.D.
Professor of Pediatrics and Medicine, Adolescent Medicine, Children's
 Hospital Medical Center, Cincinnati
Former president, Society for Adolescent Medicine

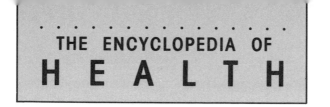

THE ENCYCLOPEDIA OF HEALTH

THE HEALTHY BODY

Dale C. Garell, M.D. · General Editor

THE ENDOCRINE SYSTEM

Marjorie Little

Introduction by C. Everett Koop, M.D., Sc.D.
former Surgeon General, U.S. Public Health Service

CHELSEA HOUSE PUBLISHERS
New York · Philadelphia

ON THE COVER Major glands of the endocrine system, illustrated by Bill Donahey.

Chelsea House Publishers
EDITOR-IN-CHIEF Nancy Toff
EXECUTIVE EDITOR Remmel T. Nunn
MANAGING EDITOR Karyn Gullen Browne
COPY CHIEF Juliann Barbato
PICTURE EDITOR Adrian G. Allen
ART DIRECTOR Maria Epes
MANUFACTURING MANAGER Gerald Levine

The Encyclopedia of Health
SENIOR EDITOR Paula Edelson

Staff for THE ENDOCRINE SYSTEM
ASSOCIATE EDITOR Kate Barrett
DEPUTY COPY CHIEF Mark Rifkin
COPY EDITOR Richard Klin
EDITORIAL ASSISTANT Leigh Hope Wood
PICTURE RESEARCHERS Sandy Jones and Bill Rice
ASSISTANT ART DIRECTOR Loraine Machlin
SENIOR DESIGNER Marjorie Zaum
DESIGN ASSISTANT Debora Smith
PRODUCTION MANAGER Joseph Romano
PRODUCTION COORDINATOR Marie Claire Cebrián

3 5 7 9 8 6 4

Library of Congress Cataloging-in-Publication Data

Little, Marjorie.
    The endocrine system/Marjorie Little.
    p. cm.—(The Encyclopedia of health. Healthy body)
    Includes bibliographical references.
    Summary: Describes the basic features of the endocrine system, the structure and function of its glands and hormones, and the causes and treatment of endocrine disorders.
    ISBN 0-7910-0016-8.
        0-7910-0456-2 (pbk.)
    1. Endocrine glands—Physiology—Juvenile literature. 2. Endocrine glands—Diseases—Juvenile literature. 3. Hormones—Physiological effect—Juvenile literature. [1. Endocrine glands. 2. Hormones.]
    I. Title. II. Series.
QP187.L534 1990
612.4—dc20
                                                                        89-25314
                                                                        CIP
                                                                        AC

CONTENTS

The goal of the ENCYCLOPEDIA OF HEALTH *is to provide general information in the ever-changing areas of physiology, psychology, and related medical issues. The titles in this series are not intended to take the place of the professional advice of a physician or other health-care professional.*

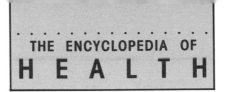

PREVENTION AND EDUCATION: THE KEYS TO GOOD HEALTH

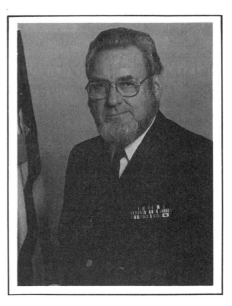

C. Everett Koop, M.D., Sc.D.
former Surgeon General,
U.S. Public Health Service

The issue of health education has received particular attention in recent years because of the presence of AIDS in the news. But our response to this particular tragedy points up a number of broader issues that doctors, public health officials, educators, and the public face. In particular, it points up the necessity for sound health education for citizens of all ages.

Over the past 25 years this country has been able to bring about dramatic declines in the death rates for heart disease, stroke, accidents, and, for people under the age of 45, cancer. Today, Americans generally eat better and take better care of themselves than ever before. Thus, with the help of modern science and technology, they have a better chance of surviving serious—even catastrophic—illnesses. That's the good news.

But, like every phonograph record, there's a flip side, and one with special significance for young adults. According to a report issued in 1979 by Dr. Julius Richmond, my predecessor as Surgeon General, Americans aged 15 to 24 had a higher death rate in 1979 than they did 20 years earlier. The causes: violent death and injury, alcohol and drug abuse, unwanted pregnancies, and sexually transmitted diseases. Adolescents are particularly vulnerable, because they are beginning to explore their own sexuality and perhaps to experiment with drugs. The need for educating young people is critical, and the price of neglect is high.

Yet even for the population as a whole, our health is still far from what it could be. Why? A 1974 Canadian government report attributed all death and disease to four broad elements: inadequacies in the health-care system, behavioral factors or unhealthy life-styles, environmental hazards, and human biological factors.

To be sure, there are diseases that are still beyond the control of even our advanced medical knowledge and techniques. And despite yearnings that are as old as the human race itself, there is no "fountain of youth" to ward off aging and death. Still, there is a solution to many of the problems that undermine sound health. In a word, that solution is prevention. Prevention, which includes health promotion and education, saves lives, improves the quality of life, and, in the long run, saves money.

In the United States, organized public health activities and preventive medicine have a long history. Important milestones include the improvement of sanitary procedures and the development of pasteurized milk in the late 19th century, and the introduction in the mid-20th century of effective vaccines against polio, measles, German measles, mumps, and other once-rampant diseases. Internationally, organized public health efforts began on a wide-scale basis with the International Sanitary Conference of 1851, to which 12 nations sent representatives. The World Health Organization, founded in 1948, continues these efforts under the aegis of the United Nations, with particular emphasis on combatting communicable diseases and the training of health-care workers.

But despite these accomplishments, much remains to be done in the field of prevention. For too long, we have had a medical care system that is science- and technology-based, focused, essentially, on illness and mortality. It is now patently obvious that both the social and the economic costs of such a system are becoming insupportable.

Implementing prevention—and its corollaries, health education and promotion—is the job of several groups of people:

First, the medical and scientific professions need to continue basic scientific research, and here we are making considerable progress. But increased concern with prevention will also have a decided impact on how primary-care doctors practice medicine. With a shift to health-based rather than morbidity-based medicine, the role of the "new physician" will include a healthy dose of patient education.

Second, practitioners of the social and behavioral sciences—psychologists, economists, city planners—along with lawyers, business leaders, and government officials—must solve the practical and ethical dilemmas confronting us: poverty, crime, civil rights, literacy, education, employment, housing, sanitation, environmental protection, health care delivery systems, and so forth. All of these issues affect public health.

Third is the public at large. We'll consider that very important group in a moment.

Fourth, and the linchpin in this effort, is the public health profession—doctors, epidemiologists, teachers—who must harness the professional expertise of the first two groups and the common sense and cooperation of the third, the public. They must define the problems statistically and qualitatively and then help us set priorities for finding the solutions.

To a very large extent, improving those statistics is the responsibility of every individual. So let's consider more specifically what the role of the individual should be and why health education is so important to that role. First, and most obviously, individuals can protect themselves from illness and injury and thus minimize their need for professional medical care. They can eat a nutritious diet, get adequate exercise, avoid tobacco, alcohol, and drugs, and take prudent steps to avoid accidents. The proverbial "apple a day keeps the doctor away" is not so far from the truth, after all.

Second, individuals should actively participate in their own medical care. They should schedule regular medical and dental checkups. Should they develop an illness or injury, they should know when to treat themselves and when to seek professional help. To gain the maximum benefit from any medical treatment that they do require, individuals must become partners in that treatment. For instance, they should understand the effects and side effects of medications. I counsel young physicians that there is no such thing as too much information when talking with patients. But the corollary is the patient must know enough about the nuts and bolts of the healing process to understand what the doctor is telling him. That is at least partially the patient's responsibility.

Education is equally necessary for us to understand the ethical and public policy issues in health care today. Sometimes individuals will encounter these issues in making decisions about their own treatment or that of family members. Other citizens may encounter them as jurors in medical malpractice cases. But we all become involved, indirectly, when we elect our public officials, from school board members to the president. Should surrogate parenting be legal? To what extent is drug testing desirable, legal, or necessary? Should there be public funding for family planning, hospitals, various types of medical research, and medical care for the indigent? How should we allocate scant technological resources, such as kidney dialysis and organ transplants? What is the proper role of government in protecting the rights of patients?

What are the broad goals of public health in the United States today? In 1980, the Public Health Service issued a report aptly entitled *Promoting Health-Preventing Disease: Objectives for the Nation.* This report expressed its goals in terms of mortality and in terms of intermediate goals in education and health improvement. It identified 15 major concerns: controlling high blood pressure; improving family planning; improving pregnancy care and infant health; increasing the rate of immunization; controlling sexually transmitted diseases; controlling the presence of toxic agents and radiation in the environment; improving occupational safety and health; preventing accidents; promoting water fluoridation and dental health; controlling infectious diseases; decreasing smoking; decreasing alcohol and drug abuse; improving nutrition; promoting physical fitness and exercise; and controlling stress and violent behavior.

For healthy adolescents and young adults (ages 15 to 24), the specific goal was a 20% reduction in deaths, with a special focus on motor vehicle injuries and alcohol and drug abuse. For adults (ages 25 to 64), the aim was 25% fewer deaths, with a concentration on heart attacks, strokes, and cancers.

Smoking is perhaps the best example of how individual behavior can have a direct impact on health. Today cigarette smoking is recognized as the most important single preventable cause of death in our society. It is responsible for more cancers and more cancer deaths than any other known agent; is a prime risk factor for heart and blood vessel disease, chronic bronchitis, and emphysema; and is a frequent cause of complications in pregnancies and of babies born prematurely, underweight, or with potentially fatal respiratory and cardiovascular problems.

Since the release of the Surgeon General's first report on smoking in 1964, the proportion of adult smokers has declined substantially, from 43% in 1965 to 30.5% in 1985. Since 1965, 37 million people have quit smoking. Although there is still much work to be done if we are to become a "smoke-free society," it is heartening to note that public health and public education efforts—such as warnings on cigarette packages and bans on broadcast advertising—have already had significant effects.

In 1835, Alexis de Tocqueville, a French visitor to America, wrote, "In America the passion for physical well-being is general." Today, as then, health and fitness are front-page items. But with the greater scientific and technological resources now available to us, we are in a far stronger position to make good health care available to everyone. And with the greater technological threats to us as we approach the 21st century, the need to do so is more urgent than ever before. Comprehensive information about basic biology, preventive medicine, medical and surgical treatments, and related ethical and public policy issues can help you arm yourself with the knowledge you need to be healthy throughout your life.

FOREWORD

Dale C. Garell, M.D.

Advances in our understanding of health and disease during the 20th century have been truly remarkable. Indeed, it could be argued that modern health care is one of the greatest accomplishments in all of human history. In the early 1900s, improvements in sanitation, water treatment, and sewage disposal reduced death rates and increased longevity. Previously untreatable illnesses can now be managed with antibiotics, immunizations, and modern surgical techniques. Discoveries in the fields of immunology, genetic diagnosis, and organ transplantation are revolutionizing the prevention and treatment of disease. Modern medicine is even making inroads against cancer and heart disease, two of the leading causes of death in the United States.

Although there is much to be proud of, medicine continues to face enormous challenges. Science has vanquished diseases such as smallpox and polio, but new killers, most notably AIDS, confront us. Moreover, we now victimize ourselves with what some have called "diseases of choice," or those brought on by drug and alcohol abuse, bad eating habits, and mismanagement of the stresses and strains of contemporary life. The very technology that is doing so much to prolong life has brought with it previously unimaginable ethical dilemmas related to issues of death and dying. The rising cost of health-care is a matter of central concern to us all. And violence in the form of automobile accidents, homicide, and suicide remain the major killers of young adults.

In the past, most people were content to leave health care and medical treatment in the hands of professionals. But since the 1960s, the consumer of medical care—that is, the patient—has assumed an increasingly central role in the management of his or her own health. There has also been a new emphasis placed on prevention: People are recognizing that their own actions can help prevent many of the conditions that have caused death and disease in the past. This accounts for the growing commitment to good nutrition and regular exercise, for the fact that more and more people are choosing not to smoke, and for a new moderation in people's drinking habits.

People want to know more about themselves and their own health. They are curious about their body: its anatomy, physiology, and biochemistry. They want to keep up with rapidly evolving medical technologies and procedures. They are willing to educate themselves about common disorders and diseases so that they can be full partners in their own health-care.

The ENCYCLOPEDIA OF HEALTH is designed to provide the basic knowledge that readers will need if they are to take significant responsibility for their own health. It is also meant to serve as a frame of reference for further study and exploration. The ENCYCLOPEDIA is divided into five subsections: The Healthy Body; The Life Cycle; Medical Disorders & Their Treatment; Psychological Disorders & Their Treatment; and Medical Issues. For each topic covered by the ENCYCLOPEDIA, we present the essential facts about the relevant biology; the symptoms, diagnosis, and treatment of common diseases and disorders; and ways in which you can prevent or reduce the severity of health problems when that is possible. The ENCYCLOPEDIA also projects what may lie ahead in the way of future treatment or prevention strategies.

The broad range of topics and issues covered in the ENCYCLOPEDIA reflects the fact that human health encompasses physical, psychological, social, environmental, and spiritual well-being. Just as the mind and the body are inextricably linked, so, too, is the individual an integral part of the wider world that comprises his or her family, society, and environment. To discuss health in its broadest aspect it is necessary to explore the many ways in which it is connected to such fields as law, social science, public policy, economics, and even religion. And so, the ENCYCLOPEDIA is meant to be a bridge between science, medical technology, the world at large, and you. I hope that it will inspire you to pursue in greater depth particular areas of interest, and that you will take advantage of the suggestions for further reading and the lists of resources and organizations that can provide additional information.

AUTHOR'S
PREFACE

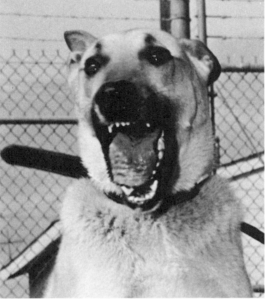

A stimulus for the fight-or-flight response

Imagine you are walking down the street. Perhaps you are thinking about a homework assignment or a movie you might want to see this weekend. Suddenly, a giant dog leaps from behind a parked car and lunges toward you. Instantly your body reacts: You breathe faster. Blood rushes to your head, and your heart beats loudly and quickly. You feel hot, and your palms are moist with sweat. Without even thinking about it, you are preparing for fight or flight. This automatic reaction to an emergency situation could save your life. It is also an instance when you can actually feel your endocrine system at work.

Beneath the surface, a complex chemical process has been set into motion: Your adrenal medulla secretes epinephrine, also known as adrenaline, into your bloodstream. As a result, your heart rate increases and pumps more oxygen into your blood. Your spleen releases more red blood cells to carry this oxygen to your muscles, and your liver secretes stored nutrients to feed them. Sympathetic neurons stimulate sweat glands in your skin to regulate the temperature of your overheated body.

This response to a stressful situation is but one example of the many ways in which the endocrine system, along with the nervous system, regulates and coordinates bodily functions. The endocrine system is comprised of nine glands and the products they secrete. The term *endocrine* derives from two Greek words, *end-* and *krinein*, meaning respectively "within" and "to separate," and describes how endocrine glands both secrete products within the glands and influence tissues separated from them.

Human bodies have two varieties of glands: *exocrine* and *en-*

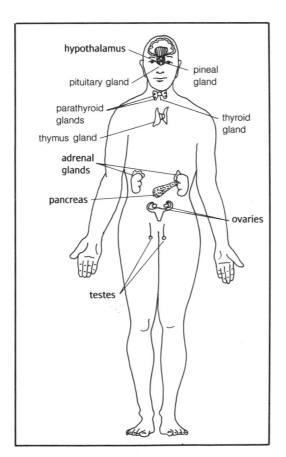

The glands of the endocrine system

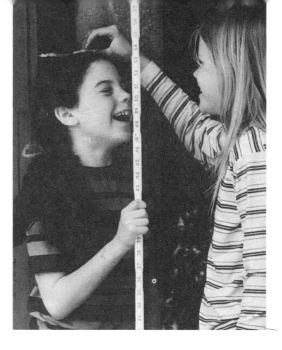

The growth process, so accelerated during childhood, is visual proof of a healthy endocrine system.

docrine. The exocrine glands have ducts or channels that direct their products to very specific locations. Sweat glands, salivary glands, and the liver are good examples. In contrast, endocrine glands produce substances that go directly into the bloodstream. They are also known as ductless glands, or glands of internal secretion. Included in this category are the pituitary, the thyroid and parathyroid glands, the thymus and pineal body, the adrenals, the pancreas, and the testes and ovaries. (Not all are agreed that the pineal body functions as a gland.)

The products of the endocrine system are called *hormones* from the Greek word *horman*, which means, "to stir up." When one is extremely scared or sexually aroused, the "exciting" or stimulating effect of hormones is apparent. Hormones play an equally important, though less visible, role in suppressing and regulating the activity of many other vital organs.

To date, scientists have identified more than 100 hormones. Each travels freely throughout the body. Some hormones affect a wide variety of cells, whereas others have a very limited range of activity. Only cells that have been programmed to react will respond to the presence of a hormone. These cells are called *target cells* and are extremely receptive. As little as one hormone cell for every million blood cells is sufficient to generate a reaction from a target cell.

The hormones of the endocrine system play a crucial role in controlling many functions of the body. They determine one's response in an emergency. They direct the complex processes of sexual maturation, which begins at puberty. They allow the human body to fight infection and feed its cells. The body must be able to monitor hormone levels and adjust production and secretion according to constantly changing needs.

A malfunction within this delicate system may result in a life-threatening disease, as in the condition of *diabetes mellitus*, the most common endocrine disorder in the United States. This illness is caused by an abnormality in the secretion of the insulin hormone. The gland responsible for the production of insulin is the pancreas, the only gland with both exocrine and endocrine functions. As an exocrine gland, it produces secretions that go directly by ducts to the intestine to aid digestion. As an endocrine gland, it contains many hundreds of thousands of microscopic cells known as the *islets of Langerhans*. These manufacture a variety of hormones, including *insulin*.

Without sufficient insulin, cells are unable to metabolize or utilize glucose, the body's basic fuel. The condition of diabetes mellitus can also occur when insulin is available but the body is unable to utilize it or when the insulin the body secretes is abnormal. If a severe case of any of these forms of diabetes goes untreated, the body will not receive sufficient nutrition, and eventually the nervous system will be affected. The patient may then fall into an irreversible diabetic coma.

The discovery of insulin in the 1920s is considered by many to be the greatest advance in endocrinology in the 20th century. Without insulin, doctors had very little they could offer as treatment to diabetic patients whose symptoms stemmed from lack of insulin. Now, through replacement therapy, most of these people can live a normal life span.

Immediate, short-term, long-term, cyclical, and lifelong processes depend on the proper functioning of the endocrine system. The chapters that follow will explain how this pivotal system functions, what happens when something goes wrong, and what physicians know, or do not know, about treating different types of imbalances. Learning about the endocrine system will provide information on how people mature, how they deal with stress, how they reproduce, and how they differ from one another.

•　　　•　　　•　　　•

CHAPTER 1

AN OVERVIEW OF THE SYSTEM

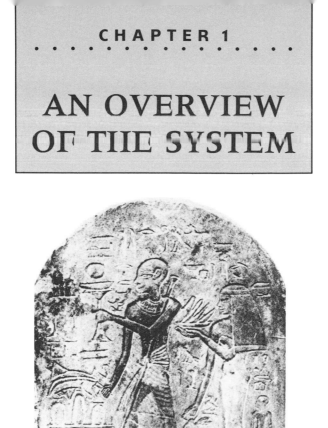

An ancient Egyptian depiction of a woman doctor

Endocrinology is the branch of medical science that explores the structure of the endocrine glands and the hormones they secrete. Although some observations of this bodily system date back to ancient times, most research on the endocrine system did not occur until the modern era.

In the 3rd century B.C., the ancient Greek philosopher and scientist Aristotle observed the varying effects of castration on calves and bulls, and long before, in the ancient civilizations of

Egypt and China, human behavioral changes resulting from removal of the testes were common knowledge. (Castration was practiced in both these civilizations to produce a servile class of men called eunuchs.) It was not really until the 17th century, however, that scientists gained empirical knowledge of the system of glands and their hormonal functions.

THREE CENTURIES OF DISCOVERY

One of the first important steps regarding physiological exploration occurred in 17th-century England, when the scientist Thomas Wharton disproved the commonly held belief that the brain was a gland that secreted mucus. Wharton was also the first to recognize the difference between the ductless and ductile glands, which differentiates the endocrine and exocrine systems.

The 17th century also saw the first observations concerning the existence of hormones. In the 1690s, Fredrik Ruysch, a well-respected Dutch scientist, claimed that the thyroid gland "poured

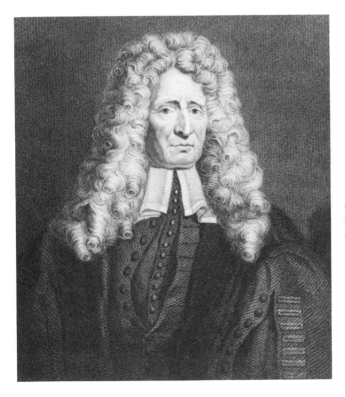

The Dutch scientist Fredrik Ruysch surmised that the thyroid excreted substances into the blood.

important substances into the blood stream." Thirty years earlier, Theophile Bordeu, a Frenchman regarded by many as the founder of endocrinology, had declared that some parts of the body gave off "emanations" that had dramatic effects on other parts of the body.

Toward the end of the 18th century, doctors began to associate a swollen neck, staring, or "bug" eyes, a racing pulse, and uncontrollable muscle tremors with a swollen thyroid gland. Some patients had such distended glands that it appeared as if huge disfiguring growths were attempting to burst from the front of their necks. This enlargement is called a toxic goiter, which is now known to be caused by excess production of the thyroid hormone.

The earliest information about the endocrine system was first obtained from the study of patients with diseased glands. In 1849, British scientist Thomas Addison reported on 11 patients who exhibited the symptoms of anemia: their blood lacked sufficient hemoglobin, (the compound in red blood cells that carries oxygen to all the cells of the body); they frequently felt faint or lethargic; they had weak hearts; and their skin was a sickly, gray color. They died soon after he examined them. Addison performed autopsies on all of these patients and discovered that every one of them had diseased *adrenal glands*. Addison named the disease "melasma suprarenale," but it was later changed to Addison's disease. (President John F. Kennedy suffered from this disorder, but his doctors were able to control its effects.)

The same year Addison made his discoveries, A. A. Berthold, a German doctor, released the results of his experiments with six young male chickens, providing the first experimental proof of the existence and functioning of hormones. Berthold had castrated four of the chickens. Two of these were left to develop without their testes. He transplanted the testes of two other chickens back into their bodies, but in a distant location from where the testes had originated. The two chickens who were not castrated grew into normal roosters, sprouting the combs, wattles, and feathers of adult male birds. In contrast, the two chickens who developed without their testes never developed adult male characteristics; their combs atrophied or shrunk. This provided the first documented proof of a hormonal deficiency.

What is equally interesting, however, is that the two birds who

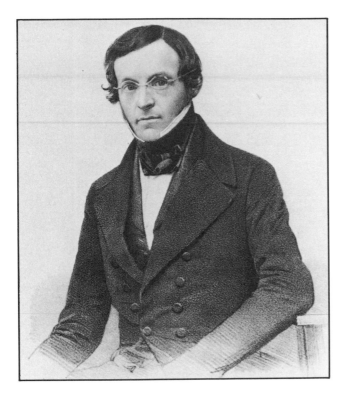

In 1849, the German doctor A. A. Berthold observed the function of testes in roosters.

had their testes removed and then relocated also developed into normal, sexually mature roosters. This offered evidence that hormones travel freely through the bloodstream and that where they originate is not crucial to how they function, as long as they are directly connected to the circulatory system.

Over the last hundred years medical researchers have greatly advanced this early exploration of the endocrine system. What follows is an overview of how this system functions.

HOW THE SYSTEM WORKS

Whereas the respiratory system supplies oxygen to the blood, and the cardiovascular system controls the circulation of blood throughout the body, the endocrine system regulates the flow of hormones in the bloodstream. These hormones play a central role in making humans what they are; they determine rate of growth and maturation and directly influence intelligence, physical agility, and sexual drives.

Production and Secretion of Hormones

The endocrine system, along with the nervous system, controls the production and secretion of hormones. Scientists once believed that the endocrine system functioned independently of the nervous system, but they now recognize the interdependence of these two regulatory systems.

The endocrine and nervous systems both regulate bodily activities, but they do so in fundamentally different ways. Endocrine glands send chemical messengers through the bloodstream, whereas the nervous system depends on electrical rather than chemical signals and sends them along a network of specialized cells called neurons. There are exceptions to these rules, however: Some neurons secrete chemicals called neurohormones, which function much like normal hormones, and some endocrine glands secrete hormones that directly influence the activity of the nervous system. Therefore, despite the basic distinction between the functioning of the two systems, they remain intertwined to a great degree.

Working in conjunction, then, the endocrine system and the nervous system provide continual information, or *feedback*,

This illustration shows how negative and positive feedback systems regulate the production of hormones.

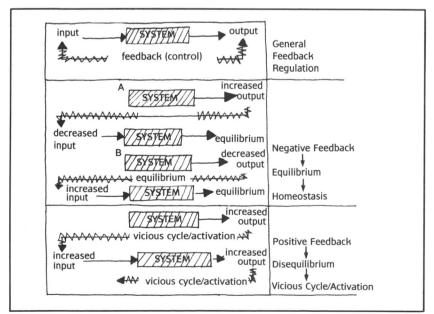

21

about the amount of hormones that are circulating through the bloodstream. If the level of any hormone in the blood is too low, the systems will signal the appropriate gland. If the hormone level is too high, another set of signals will shut down glandular production. This is known as *negative feedback* control. It gets this name because it works on the principle of reversing any excess or deficit that exists. It is through negative feedback that most hormone levels are regulated, much like water in a tank: When the tank is low, the fill mechanism will automatically allow water to enter. Once the tank is full, the fill mechanism shuts off the supply of water.

A few hormones, however, operate on a *positive feedback* principle. In this case, the presence of one hormone stimulates the production and secretion of another. The menstrual cycle in females provides an excellent example. Each month one of the ovaries produces an egg. As the egg grows, the ovary releases the hormone *estrogen* into the bloodstream. The rise in estrogen triggers the pituitary gland to release an additional sex hormone called LH, which stands for luteinizing hormone. In turn, LH stimulates the ovary to release the mature egg into the nearby oviduct. This final process, called *ovulation*, is the result of a chain reaction that began with a chemical message from the endocrine system.

Hormonal Reception

How do hormones know where to go to find appropriate target cells? Actually, they do not. They are simply carried along in the bloodstream, where they will eventually come into contact with cells that are programmed to respond to their presence. It is up to these target cells to react as the hormones pass by. They do this through a mechanism called a *receptor*. Essentially a large protein molecule, a receptor is continually on the lookout for a specific type of chemical, in this case a specific hormone; when one passes by, the receptor recognizes it, attracts it, and captures it. Because hormones are normally produced in minute quantities, receptors must be extremely sensitive and efficient. This sensitivity is the most crucial factor for the expression of hormonal activity. If receptor sites break down, hormones will not

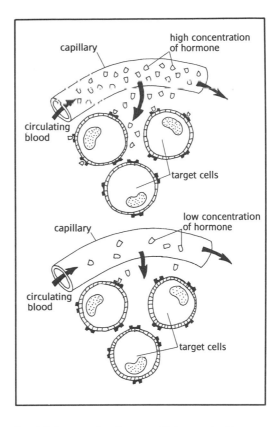

Hormones are diffused from the blood through the walls of the capillaries into intermediary spaces, where target cells receive them. The capillaries diffuse more or less hormone, depending on its concentration in the blood.

be able to affect target cells. This results in conditions similar to those caused by the lack of adequate hormone production.

Most hormones—insulin, for example—are too large to enter a target cell. They attach themselves to an external receptor and use it to transmit a message to the cell's interior. Some hormones, such as *testosterone*, a male sex hormone, are small enough to penetrate the cell's surface. They stimulate internal receptors and travel into the nucleus. Here, they activate specific genes that carry out the hormone's function.

Then the action begins. The target cells respond. The exact nature of their response depends on the type of cell. Muscle cells may increase or decrease contraction. *Epithelial cells*, which are found in skin surfaces and in the walls of many internal organs, alter the rate at which liquids are allowed to pass through them. Gland cells function as a group to secrete more or less of the chemicals they produce. This allows the body to constantly adjust levels of salt and water in its tissues as well as to regulate the amount of sugar in the blood and the amount of salt in sweat.

All of these constant changes help the body maintain a vital chemical balance.

After the hormone has contacted its receptor cell, the continued existence of the hormone is no longer required, and the hormone is either excreted from the circulatory system by the kidneys or degraded by enzymes within the blood, liver, kidney, lungs, or target tissues. If it were not, its biological effect would continue indefinitely as long as the hormone survived.

Endocrinologists can determine hormone levels by studying not only how quickly the glands produce hormones but also how quickly hormones are destroyed. They do this by measuring how long it takes half a dose of a hormone to leave the circulatory system. This period of time, known as a half-life, is a means of predicting the rate at which hormones are eliminated from the body. (The total elimination of a substance is not a useful gauge because it is dramatically influenced by its starting concentration.) This measurement is known as the *metabolic clearance rate*. It measures the elimination of hormone molecules by both the liver and kidneys. It also takes into account the hormones that target cells ingest and destroy. The metabolic clearance rate can play a significant role in determining the frequency of drug administration.

In brief, hormonal communication can be measured in seven overall stages: It begins with signals from the nervous system or endocrine system that stimulate hormonal production. This is followed by the second and third stages, which involve secretion and delivery to target cells. During the fourth stage the cell receptors recognize the hormone, and in stage five, target cells respond. Once a hormone has performed its function, it enters stage six and is destroyed or degraded. Signaling the elimination of hormone cells is the final stage of communication.

MALFUNCTION

About 10% of the population of most developed nations will experience some form of endocrine disorder. Most endocrine system disorders involve a glandular problem, such as a tumor, which results in either overproduction (hyperfunction) or underproduction (hypofunction) of hormones.

In the case of the thyroid gland, *hyperthyroidism* and *hypothyroidism* can cause gland enlargement or additional tumors. Toxic goiters provide a very visual symptom of *hyperthyroidism*, or excess hormone production by the thyroid gland. Simple goiters result from *hypothyroidism*, a condition that is primarily caused by a lack of iodine in the diet and occurs very rarely today because iodine is now a common ingredient in table salt.

In addition to the overproduction or underproduction of hormones, endocrine system disorders may involve an enhancement or diminishment in the sensitivity of target cells; genetic defects that may cause abnormalities in hormone synthesis; and tumors, cysts, or infections of endocrine glands.

Treatment for the underproduction, or hypofunction, of hormones generally involves simply administering the missing hormones directly into the bloodstream, though in some cases a different hormone or a totally separate chemical may be substi-

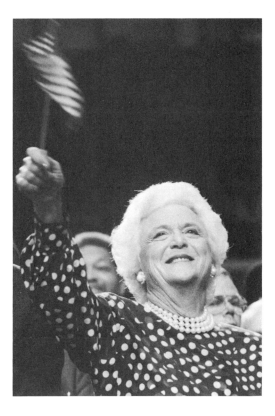

First Lady Barbara Bush, who suffers from hypothyroidism, at the Republican National Convention in 1988.

tuted. Treatment for the overproduction, or hyperfunction, of hormones may take a variety of approaches. If a tumor is causing a gland to hyperfunction, the tumor will usually be removed. In other cases, drugs are prescribed that can block the production of specific hormones.

In the chapters that follow, the major organs of the endocrine system will be described. Hormones, the key players of this system, will be presented, and their lifelong, wide-ranging influence will be examined.

•   •   •   •

CHAPTER 2

THE PITUITARY GLAND

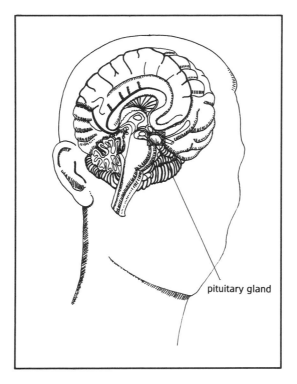

The pituitary gland serves so many vital functions that it has been called the master gland.

Look in the mirror and imagine a line going from the bridge of your nose straight back, deep into the center of your head. If you were able to see inside yourself, you would find a tiny organ there about the size of a pinto bean. It is surrounded by bone and appears to be hanging from the base of the brain. This is your pituitary gland. Although one of the smallest endocrine glands, this organ has been known throughout history as the master gland. It retains this title for several reasons: First, it is a primary link between the nervous system and the endocrine system. Second, it produces and releases a wide variety of hormones that control the functioning of other endocrine glands. And finally, it directs some fundamental life processes. The pituitary determines how tall you will grow and how early you will embark on the journey through puberty.

THE MASTER'S MASTER

The pituitary gland is comprised of two distinct segments. The front part is called the *anterior lobe*; the section closer to the back of the skull is the *posterior lobe*. Although both lobes together are only about the size of a small acorn, each functions as an independent gland with its own distinct activities. The posterior lobe makes up approximately 25% of the entire gland. It stores and secretes two hormones manufactured in a part of the brain called the *hypothalamus*. The anterior lobe comprises the remaining 75% of the pituitary.

Both sections of the pituitary are directly connected to, and controlled by, the hypothalamus, a section of the brain control-

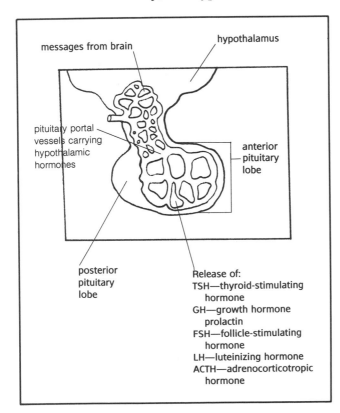

messages from brain

hypothalamus

pituitary portal vessels carrying hypothalamic hormones

anterior pituitary lobe

posterior pituitary lobe

Release of:
TSH—thyroid-stimulating hormone
GH—growth hormone
prolactin
FSH—follicle-stimulating hormone
LH—luteinizing hormone
ACTH—adrenocorticotropic hormone

The hypothalamus enables the anterior pituitary to release hormones that relay crucial information between the brain and body.

ling the basic survival processes of hunger, thirst, sexual reproduction, and self-defense. A stem containing both neurons and
small blood vessels connects the pituitary gland with the hypothalamus. Thus, the hypothalamus communicates with the pituitary in two ways: by nerve impulses and by chemical
messengers. The anterior pituitary receives instructions from the
hypothalamus in the form of *releasing hormones*. These chemical
messengers produced by the hypothalamus then travel through
the blood. A special network of vessels directs this blood through
the anterior pituitary before it returns to the heart. In contrast,
the posterior pituitary receives its messages through neural tissue
and is controlled by nerve impulses.

All information that enters the brain must pass through the
hypothalamus. The pituitary gland plays a key role in the ability
of the hypothalamus to act on this information and initiate the
proper physical response.

A CALL TO ACTION

The major function of the anterior pituitary is *tropic*. This does
not, however, have anything to do with climate, palm trees, or
exotic fruits. In this case, the suffix *-tropic* is used to indicate
hormones that affect other glands and organs. The anterior pituitary produces six crucial tropic hormones:

1. Growth hormone (GH) or somatotropic hormone.

2. Thyroid-stimulating hormone (TSH) or thyrotropic hormone.

3. Adrenocorticotropic hormone (ACTH).

4. Follicle-stimulating hormone (FSH), a gonadotropic hormone.

5. Luteinizing hormone (LH), a gonadotropic hormone.

6. Prolactin or lactotropic hormone (LTH).

These hormones determine the size of both the glands and
organs they affect as well as the production and secretion of these
glands' hormonal products. And, if the anterior lobe secretes an
abnormal amount of one hormone or another, the results are
often plainly visible.

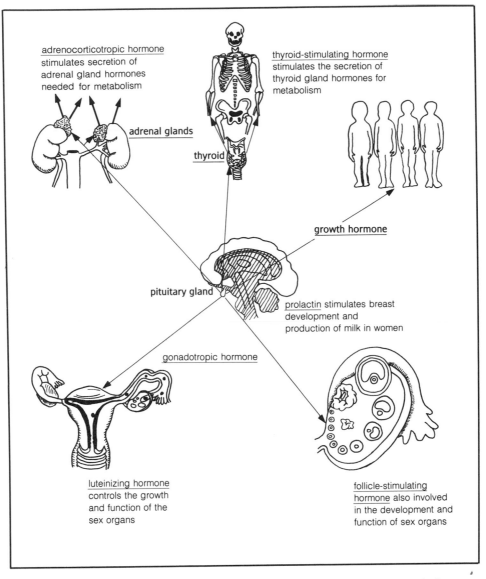

The hormones that the pituitary releases influence the body's metabolism and development.

A Growing Concern

On June 18, 1955, Sandy Allen was born in Shelbyville, Indiana. Soon after her birth, her parents noticed that she seemed to be growing faster than normal—much faster. She continued to grow rapidly as a child and as a teenager. By the time Allen was 22 years old, she measured 7 feet 7¼ inches tall. This makes her the tallest living woman in the world, according to the 1989 *Guinness Book of World Records*.

Of course, giantism is nothing new. Written documentation exists from centuries ago. One particularly interesting, though grisly, case, dating from the 18th century, concerns the history of a subject named O'Brien, "the Irish Giant." At the age of 22, O'Brien's height was 8 feet 4 inches. Apparently O'Brien's size came to the attention of a well-respected scientist by the name of John Hunter. Hunter became obsessed with obtaining O'Brien's body once the Irish Giant died. Hunter intended to boil the corpse until only its impressive skeleton remained. O'Brien was not nearly so keen on this plan.

In 1783, O'Brien, on his deathbed, bribed some local fishermen to take his body to the middle of the Irish Channel, attach weights to it, and drop it overboard. Unfortunately for O'Brien, but possibly of benefit to the medical community, Hunter found out and offered the fishermen a larger bribe to deliver the body to him. O'Brien's skeleton, as well as the kettle in which it was prepared, are now part of the collection of the Museum of the Royal College of Surgeons.

Allen and O'Brien were both affected by an overproduction of growth hormone (GH). This hormone has the crucial regulatory

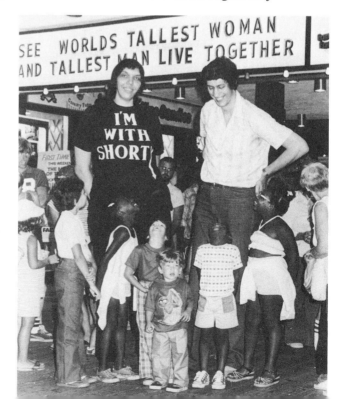

Chris Greener (right) is a half inch shorter than Sandy Allen (left), who at seven feet seven inches is the world's tallest woman. Their immense height is due to an overproduction of growth hormone.

function of stimulating growth until maturity. It is particularly influential in determining the length of bones. The level of growth hormone in plasma is at its highest level at birth. In adolescence, the production rate of growth hormone is nearly double the rate during prepuberty. But the anterior lobe continues to secrete GH every day—even in adults—and is at its busiest during the first hour and a half of a person's sleep, when it secretes almost half of its daily amount.

Medical problems caused by inappropriate levels of growth hormone are the most frequent symptoms of either a hyperactive or a hypoactive pituitary gland. In children, an excessive secretion of GH results in *giantism*. In adults, whose long bones are no longer capable of lengthening, a condition known as *acromegaly* occurs. Cartilage in the face, hands, and feet begins to grow. Bones thicken. Sinuses enlarge and the jaw widens and protrudes. The face and appendages take on a thick appearance. Hats, rings, and shoes become too tight to wear. Acromegaly most commonly occurs in people in their thirties and forties; and approximately 300 new cases are diagnosed each year.

The most frequent cause of overproduction of growth hormone is a tumor on the pituitary gland. Surgery can remove the growth, but although this effectively eliminates the production of excessive GH, it usually also shuts down the production of other crucial pituitary hormones. Patients must take replacement hormones for the rest of their life.

Dwarfism

Some people suffer from the opposite condition, called *dwarfism*, which is caused by an underproduction of growth hormone. (In about one-third of these cases the only reduced hormone is GH, whereas in two-thirds of the cases other anterior pituitary hormones aside from GH are lacking.)

Earlier civilizations often honored dwarfs for their wisdom and wit. Many noble families even adopted one or more dwarfs and bestowed special privileges upon them. Roman emperors were known to include dwarfs in their courts. Aesop, the Greek whose fables are still told today, is perhaps the best-known dwarf in history. Peter the Great of Russia sponsored many dwarfs, and

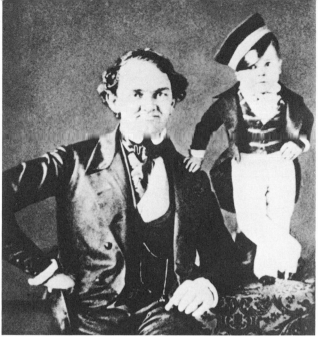

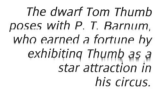

The dwarf Tom Thumb poses with P. T. Barnum, who earned a fortune by exhibiting Thumb as a star attraction in his circus.

in Spain and England, royal leaders commissioned leading artists to paint portraits of their dwarfs.

Unfortunately, however, most adults of diminished stature have suffered rather than benefited from their small size. Sideshows and circuses have exploited dwarfs for centuries. The most famous of these dwarfs was Tom Thumb, who was a star attraction of Barnum's Circus. Tom was born in Bridgeport, Connecticut, in January 1832. At the age of 5 months and at the height of 21 inches, he stopped growing. Barnum exhibited Tom throughout Europe, and both he and Tom amassed considerable fortunes. The shortest man in the world today is Nelson de la Rosa of the Dominican Republic. Mr. de la Rosa stopped growing at 28.3 inches.

Unless they receive treatment as children, people who suffer from dwarfism will never achieve adult size. Although immature in size, those who suffer from chronic hyposecretion of GH are as intellectually capable as anyone of normal height; in contrast, dwarfism caused by hyposecretion of thyroid hormones, which also affects the brain's functioning, is also marked by mental impairment.

Fortunately, recent medical and technological advances offer help to children who have a growth hormone deficiency. Parents and pediatricians should be aware of children whose growth rate is significantly below normal. These children are often no taller than children two or more years younger than they. If doctors suspect that there is a lack of GH, they can administer special tests that use a variety of growth hormone stimulants. If these substances do not affect levels of GH in the circulation, pituitary dwarfism may be diagnosed. In these cases, GH replacement will allow the children to achieve a normal adult height. This treatment should be used only when an experienced endocrinologist has determined that the body is lacking GH and has administered tests to prove it. The attending physician must then monitor treatment with extreme care.

In the past, growth hormone was very difficult to obtain. The only source was the pituitary glands of deceased people. This supplied only enough growth hormone to treat 700 children each year. But advances in biotechnology during the 1980s have led to the production of synthetic growth hormone. This should enable doctors to have an unlimited and extremely pure supply available to them in the very near future.

DIRECTING THE THYROID

As its name would imply, thyroid-stimulating hormone (TSH) plays a key role in the proper functioning of the thyroid gland. Without TSH, the thyroid gland will atrophy and cease to function. TSH acts as a conductor, directing and coordinating the thyroid's many activities: It instructs the gland to gather and store iodine from the blood, to use this iodine in the synthesis of hormones, and to release these hormones in proper quantities when appropriate. If there is not enough iodine available, additional TSH will be released, which will direct the thyroid gland to enlarge and take better advantage of what little iodine is present.

This condition was once thought to be a sign of beauty, for in its early stages the slightly bulging gland produces a very smooth throat. But unless it is corrected, the thyroid gland enlarges considerably, resulting in a goiter, which is an obvious and unsightly symptom of a thyroid disorder. Fortunately, iodine deficiencies are readily diagnosed and treated, and this type of simple goiter has become a rarity today.

The control TSH has over the thyroid gland provides an excellent example of a negative feedback loop. The hypothalamus

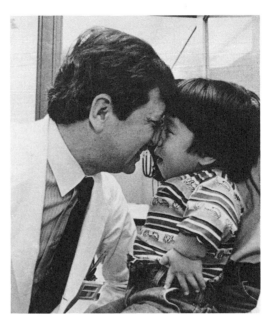

Three-year-old Benji DuGoff with Steven Kopits, an orthopedic surgeon at Johns Hopkins Hospital. Thanks to Dr. Kopits's innovative techniques, Benji, who suffers from dwarfism, can walk.

produces a releasing factor known by its full name as *thyroid-stimulating hormone releasing factor (TSH-RF)*. The anterior pituitary tissue has receptors for TSH-RF. In the presence of this hormone, the anterior pituitary produces and releases TSH into the bloodstream. The TSH reaches the thyroid gland and then stimulates it to begin synthesizing and releasing its hormones into the circulation. Signals are sent to the brain as thyroid hormone levels rise, and production of TSH is cut back until additional thyroid hormones are needed.

CONTROLLING THE ADRENAL GLANDS

Adrenocorticotropic hormone (ACTH) is the anterior pituitary hormone that directs the adrenal glands, whose function is essential to life. In a manner very similar to TSH, a delicate feedback mechanism controls levels of ACTH. The hypothalamus produces an ACTH-releasing factor that stimulates ACTH secretion from the pituitary into the bloodstream. Specially programmed receptors on the adrenal glands then pick up the ACTH. These receptors also send signals to the cell's nucleus to begin producing and secreting adrenal hormones. The hormones are released into the circulatory system, and their presence is communicated to the brain.

ACTH also helps to regulate the metabolism. These hormones include glucocorticoids, which help control the body's metabolism; mineralocorticoids, involved in regulating the amount of water in the body; and progesterone, a hormone crucial to reproduction because it prepares the uterus for the reception and preparation of a fertilized ovum.

Like many other hormones, ACTH is secreted in a *circadian pattern*, a period of time approximating 24 hours. Each person has his or her own internal circadian rhythm, which determines how much sleep that person needs, when he or she is most alert, and when he or she likes to eat. Disruptions of this rhythm can affect biological functions as well as moods and intellectual ability. Jet lag after a long flight across several time zones is probably the result of a disruption of the circadian pattern. For most people, ACTH is at its highest blood levels in the early morning. The adrenals are crucial to how well people handle stress, how rapidly they act and react, and whether or not they start the day with a boost of energy.

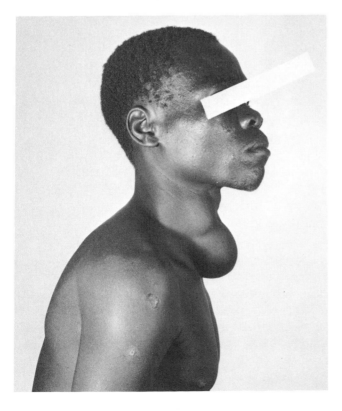

This protrusive goiter is symptomatic of hypothyroid disorder. The thyroid has enlarged to compensate for an iodine deficiency due to a poor diet.

GONADOTROPIC HORMONES

The gonadotropic hormones are appropriately named for their target organs—the gonads, or sex organs. There are two main gonadotropic hormones: follicle-stimulating hormone (FSH) and luteinizing hormone (LH). Both do double duty. They control the secretion of sex hormones and the production of mature sperm and eggs.

Although the growing fetus has high levels of FSH and LH, infants and small children produce very little. Then, however, comes puberty. Sexual maturation begins for girls at an average age of 12½ and 1 or 2 years later for boys.

Signals for the production of FSH and LH by the pituitary are also initiated in the hypothalamus. No one is absolutely certain how the hypothalamus determines when to begin stimulating the release of gonadotropins. There is, however, a definite correlation between the onset of puberty and the maturation of bones. A look at any grade school class will confirm that girls generally grow faster than boys. This discrepancy probably relates to the tendency for girls to enter puberty before boys.

The testes, or male sex organs, are under the control of both FSH, which promotes the production of sperm, and LH, which stimulates the production of *testosterone*. Although this hormone is often called the male sex hormone, this is not entirely true. LH also stimulates women's adrenal glands and ovaries to produce a small quantity of testosterone. Similarly, estrogen, labeled the female sex hormone, is produced not only in women's ovaries but also, in smaller quantities, by the adrenal glands and testes. When it comes to sex hormones, it is a question of quantity, not exclusion.

From the onset of puberty, males continuously secrete testosterone to ensure the production of mature sperm. These hormone levels are directed by a negative feedback mechanism linking the brain, the pituitary, and the body.

In females, sex hormone secretions are also directed by the release of gonadotropic hormones, but levels are cyclical rather than constant. Each cycle produces and releases only one mature egg. The length of this cycle, known as the menstrual cycle, averages 28 days. FSH levels peak at the time of ovulation. Both

FSH and LH have to be present in the blood for the ovaries to produce estrogen.

A WORD ABOUT PROLACTIN

The sixth anterior pituitary hormone discovered so far is prolactin, or lactotropic hormone. Prolactin stimulates the production of milk in the mammary glands. Of course, this normally occurs only in females who have just given birth. At this time, a complex array of hormones signals the hypothalamus to begin releasing prolactin. Many researchers believe that a prolactin-inhibiting factor (PIF) which helps to prevent untimely lactation also exists. A decline in PIF following the birth of a child is thought to temper its inhibition.

Although nursing infants are interested in only one thing—getting fed, as they suckle and empty their mothers' milk-laden breasts—they are also actually stimulating the continued production of prolactin, both maintaining an immediate, steady supply of mother's milk and securing their next meal.

Although an infrequent occurrence, an oversupply of prolactin may result in an abnormally high production of breast milk and the prevention of menstruation.

THE POSTERIOR PITUITARY

The posterior pituitary secretes two hormones: oxytocin (OT) and antidiuretic hormone (ADH). Neither of these, however, is manufactured there. Both are actually products of the hypothalamus.

Oxytocin

The hypothalamus produces oxytocin and ADH and directs them to the posterior pituitary, where they are separately stored in membrane-bound granules. Release of these hormones is totally dependent upon nerve impulses from the hypothalamus to the posterior pituitary.

In women, oxytocin works in conjunction with prolactin in providing milk to nursing infants. Oxytocin stimulates contraction of the milk ducts within the breasts, which helps eject the

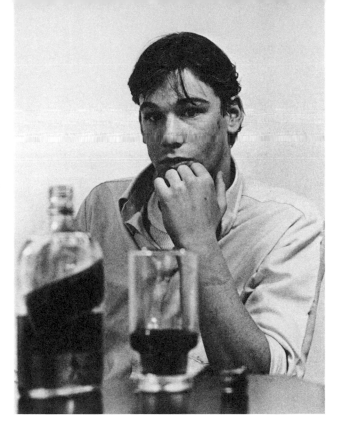

Alcohol abuse has immediate consequences and may do long-term damage to bodily functions such as reproduction.

milk. This is known as the *letdown reflex*. It also has an important function in stimulating contractions of the uterus during labor. Therapeutically, oxytocin is used to induce labor and also to stop uterine bleeding. It is not clear what role, if any, oxytocin plays in men.

Antidiuretic Hormone

The main job of antidiuretic hormone (ADH), also known as vasopressin, is water conservation. By helping the kidneys to conserve water, ADH maintains proper fluid levels in the body. As water passes through the tubules in the kidneys, it can either be reabsorbed by the body or excreted as urine. Water is reabsorbed at the proper level when there is a sufficient amount of ADH present.

If ADH secretions are too low, a disorder called *diabetes insipidus* can occur. (This is not to be confused with the much more common diabetes mellitus, which will be discussed in

Chapter 5.) The most common symptom associated with diabetes insipidus is the excretion of enormous quantities of urine—frequently as much as 10 quarts a day. This is not only a great inconvenience but can also readily lead to dehydration. Fortunately, diabetes insipidus is generally treatable with antidiuretic hormone replacement.

Alcohol is one of many factors that can depress the secretion of ADH. Often people who have had too much to drink find themselves having to urinate frequently and wake up "dying of thirst." They have temporarily dehydrated themselves by upsetting their hormonal balance. Pain, sleep, exercise, nicotine, barbiturates, and morphine are just a few of the things that have the opposite effect of increasing the production and release of ADH.

The pituitary gland plays a principal role in determining how tall a child will grow, when a girl will start to menstruate, and whether or not a man and a woman can conceive a child; and an imbalance in its secretion may influence the body's ability to metabolize food, nurse an infant, or even to get out of bed in the morning. It has certainly earned its title of the master gland; its unimpressive size belies its tremendous significance to human life.

•   •   •   •

CHAPTER 3

THE THYROID AND PARATHYROID

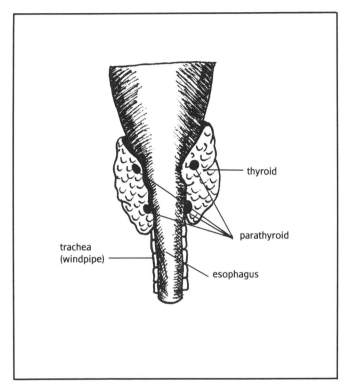

Rear view of thyroid

Take a swallow and you will feel the bulge in the front of your neck move up and down. This is your Adam's apple, a mass of tough, connective tissue that protects your voice box. Directly beneath it is your thyroid gland, the largest endocrine organ in the system. Of course, in this case "largest" is still fairly small, a normal thyroid gland weighing no more than an ounce. It looks like a reddish purple butterfly that has made a perfect landing. Its two wings, or lobes, lie fully extended on either side of the windpipe. The lobes are connected by a narrow band called the *isthmus.* Because of its location, many blood vessels pass through the thyroid, giving it its rich color and providing rapid delivery service of thyroid hormones throughout the body.

The thyroid is the body's accelerator. It determines how fast and how efficiently people digest the food they eat. Through a complicated series of processes, humans are able to ingest food and convert it into the nutrients and energy needed for survival. This combination of events is known as the body's *metabolism.* It has a lot to do with whether a person feels active, antsy, or sluggish; whether someone is generally comfortable, cold all the time, or burning up; and whether or not a person can get away with eating that extra piece of pie without gaining an ounce.

By setting the rate of metabolism, thyroid hormones play a crucial role in protein synthesis and oxygen consumption. These hormones also affect the development of the central nervous system, accelerate growth in small children, and influence the adrenal and pancreatic hormones.

You might have the impression that the thyroid gland is one organ you cannot live without. Fortunately, this is not the case. Effective replacement therapy now exists to remedy the hypoactive thyroid, and safe techniques are widely used to disarm the hyperactive one. A malfunctioning thyroid is not uncommon. As many as 20% of the people in the United States may suffer from some form of thyroid disorder in their life, and women are 5 to 9 times as likely to experience thyroid problems as men.

In ancient Roman times, a hyperactive thyroid not only created serious medical problems for many women but also had disastrous social consequences. The Romans recognized that a frequent consequence of pregnancy was a slightly enlarged thyroid gland. They took their observations one step further and incorporated a test of virginity into Roman law, based upon the measurement of the circumference of the neck. Pity the poor young girls who were highly virtuous but slightly hyperthyroid.

FUELING THE SYSTEM

Triiodothyronine and *thyroxine*, also known respectively as T3 and T4, are the thyroid hormones that regulate the metabolism. They are produced and stored in the thyroid gland. Generally, at

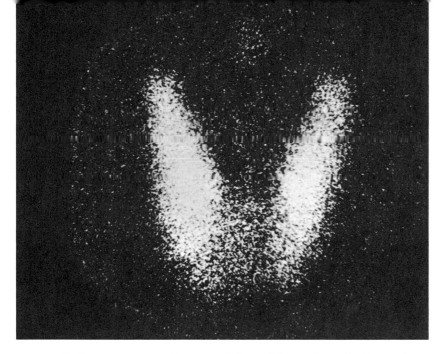

A magnified gamma scan of a normal thyroid (frontal view). Thyroid hormones control the body's metabolism, influence growth, and affect the development of the central nervous system.

least a one-month supply is on hand at all times. To produce T3 and T4, the body needs a sufficient supply of iodine—about two-millionths of an ounce a day. Although it does not sound hard to ingest such a tiny amount, insufficient iodine intake did cause problems in the past.

In 1920, the United States War Department published a study entitled "Defects Found in Drafted Men." Interestingly, the incidence of goiters coincided with those areas of the country having the least amount of iodine in their water supply. Areas surrounding the Great Lakes and Pacific Northwest were labeled goiter regions. Today though, iodine deficiency is very rare because of the widespread use of iodized salt.

Once in the body, iodine is absorbed by the gastrointestinal tract and delivered through the blood to the thyroid. The thyroid then uses the iodine to synthesize both T3 and T4. These two hormones appear to be almost exactly alike, except that T3 has only three molecules of iodine attached to it, whereas T4 has four. The thyroid secretes all of the T4 circulating in the body, but only about 20% of T3 originates in that gland. The other 80% of T3 is produced from T4 molecules that are stripped of 1 mol-

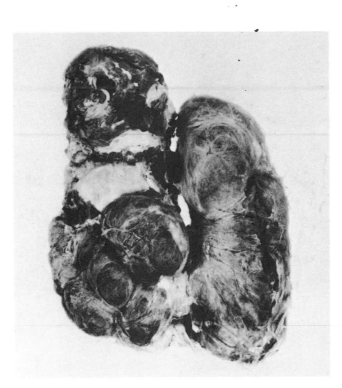

A goitrous growth attached to a thyroid. The addition of iodine to salt has made goiters a rare sight today.

ecule of iodine. This takes place primarily in the liver and kidneys. Receptors for T3 are found on the heart, the liver, the pituitary, and the kidney.

Although there are many more T4 molecules, the T3 molecules are much more powerful. In fact, scientists are still uncertain what, if any, function the T4 molecules have, other than providing a source for additional T3.

Calcitonin, the third hormone produced by the thyroid gland, plays a key role in regulating the amount of calcium circulating in the human body. Like T3 and T4, calcitonin production is regulated by a negative feedback control. When calcium levels get too high, the thyroid is signaled to speed up the production and delivery of calcitonin. It acts in opposition to the effects of calcium-stimulating hormones by preventing calcium from being *resorbed*, or leeched out of bones and into the bloodstream. It also interferes with the kidney's ability to reabsorb calcium and return it to the circulating blood.

Much more will be said about calcitonin in the following section on parathyroid glands.

MALFUNCTIONS OF THE THYROID GLAND

By its 12th week of development, the human embryo has already begun to grow a thyroid gland. In infants, *hypothyroidism,* a deficiency of thyroid hormones, is most frequently the result of the abnormal development of the fetal thyroid. Unless diagnosed within the first six months, these defects can cause irreversible complications. One of the most frequent is *cretinism.* The most obvious symptoms of infantile hypothyroidism are mental retardation and dwarfism. Because there is a lack of thyroid hormones, neither the brain nor the skeleton of the child matures. Cretins are also often retarded in their sexual development. As they get older, they exhibit a swollen face, an enlarged head, a flat nose, and widely separated eyes.

Most doctors perform routine diagnostic tests for hypothyroidism at birth. If an infant is found to have very high levels of TSH (the thyroid-stimulating hormone) in its blood but very low levels of T4, treatment is indicated. Fortunately, drug therapy to replace the missing hormones is readily available and generally safe, so that if caught early this condition and its accompanying mental retardation can be prevented.

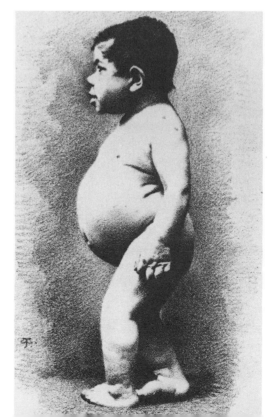

A two-year-old male cretin, 1896. If left untreated, infantile hypothyroidism may cause mental retardation and dwarfism.

Adult Hypothyroidism

The clinical name for adult hypothyroidism is myxedema. Symptomatic of this condition, which is caused by a lack of thyroid hormones, is a general retardation of bodily functions. Mental processes and speech slow down. Body temperature decreases, and sensitivity to cold escalates. The face becomes swollen and puffy. Skin may become yellow as vitamin A synthesis is impaired. Weight increases while sexual drive decreases. Menstrual periods can be extremely heavy and long. Other symptoms include backache, swollen muscles, and constipation. This slowdown can have some dramatic effects: Women can become infertile and men impotent.

The most common treatment for adult hypothyroidism is a daily maintenance dose of T4. Because T4 must be converted into T3 before if becomes effective, it works more slowly than T3. This has been proved to be therapeutically beneficial, especially for patients who have heart disease. (T4 works more slowly than T3 and so is less likely to promote heart ailments.) T4 also remains in the body longer than T3. If untreated, chronic myxedema can lead to a *myxedema coma*, a far more serious condition that can be fatal.

Hyperthyroidism

An overproduction of thyroid hormones speeds up the metabolism and produces symptoms opposite from those of myxedema. An overly fast or high metabolism results in moist, flushed skin, a rapid pulse rate, a temperature increase, muscle weakness, and diarrhea. Victims are often agitated and irritable. They perspire profusely and tend to lose weight even if they eat enormous quantities of food.

The most common form of hyperthyroidism in adults is called Graves' disease, after Dr. Robert J. Graves. In 1835, Dr. Graves treated a patient who had been in a "nervous state" for three months. Noting a horseshoe tumor in the exact location of her thyroid gland, Dr. Graves correctly diagnosed that the improper functioning of the gland was responsible for his patient's exhaustion, rapid heartbeat, weight loss, and protruding eyes. Although Graves' disease is also the most common cause of

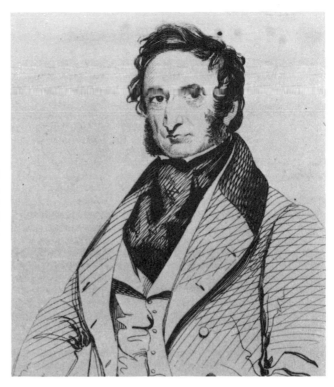

Graves' disease is named for the Irish physician Dr. Robert Graves, who was the first to diagnose this form of hyperthyroidism.

hyperthyroidism in children, its occurrence is extremely rare in children younger than five years of age.

Current medical research suggests that Graves' disease may be the result of a breakdown of the immune system. As a result, the body produces cells that attach to the receptors that are supposed to respond only to the pituitary hormone TSH. These immune cells continually activate the receptors, which in turn excite the thyroid to continue its secretion of thyroid hormones. The result is hyperproduction of these hormones.

Several other causes of hyperthyroidism are also known. One part or nodule of the entire gland may overproduce. Inflammation of the thyroid gland can cause overactivity. Tumors, although infrequent, have also been known to produce the same results. And it should not go without mention that the misuse of thyroid pills can lead to hyperthyroidism as well. The most frequent patients in this category are overweight people, frequently teenagers. They either take thyroid medication when it is not necessary or take more than the amount prescribed, thinking it will help them lose extra pounds faster.

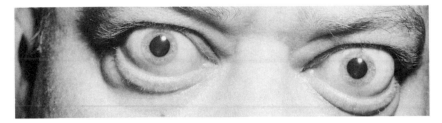

Abnormal protrusion of the eyeball, exophthalmos, is one of the symptoms of Graves' disease.

Hyperthyroidism can be treated with antithyroid drugs, radioactive iodine, or surgery. Radioactive iodine is easy to use, inexpensive, and effective. A trained physician generally prescribes it in oral form. The radioactive iodine will enter the body, go immediately to the thyroid gland, and destroy the majority of the tissue. Many physicians today prefer this type of treatment for hyperthyroidism. Long-range testing has shown that radioactive iodine therapy does not cause cancer and does not damage the sex organs. Pregnant women should avoid this type of treatment, however, for it could destroy the fetal thyroid. Surgical procedures are alternative ways of removing either some or all of the thyroid. Radioactive iodine always requires, and surgery frequently requires, a lifetime of replacement hormone therapy.

Although minor thyroid imbalances can easily be diagnosed and treated, it is estimated that in the United States alone as many as 2 million people suffer from disorders that could be avoided by a thyroid-level check during a routine physical examination.

THE PARATHYROIDS

In the 1940s, a scientist named Fuller Albright made groundbreaking discoveries about the parathyroid glands. Although at first many of his findings relied on theoretical rather than scientific proof, they initiated revolutionary advances in endocrine research. Parathyroid glands, like other endocrine glands, frequently become hyperactive when infiltrated by an *adenoma*. These are benign, or nonmalignant, tumors. Albright found that by removing these tumors he also eliminated a bone disease brought on by an overactive parathyroid gland. From this information he then hypothesized the following:

- Endocrine adenomas could also produce and secrete hormones that were similar, or identical, to those of the gland they had invaded.
- Hormone deficiency could be caused by failure of target organs to respond.
- Hormone deficiency could result from underactivity of the gland.

Albright's discoveries were but the tip of the iceberg regarding the workings of the parathyroid glands.

Some Basic Facts

There is a curious feature about the parathyroid glands: Not everyone has the same number. Most people have four. They are generally positioned toward the back of the thyroid gland and lie in stacked pairs, one pair on each side of the thyroid. It is estimated, however, that as many as 14% of the population have a fifth parathyroid, and a lesser number of people come equipped with six. Although the human body does not generally exhibit a "room for one more" attitude when it comes to organic development, the parathyroids are so tiny that extras seem to be well tolerated. A fully mature parathyroid is less than one-quarter of an inch in diameter and weighs less than a centigram. They are characteristically oval, or bean-shaped.

The main function of the parathyroid glands is to maintain the proper balance of calcium in the body through the production and secretion of parathyroid hormone. The glands have two types of cells: *Chief* cells, which supply the body with parathyroid hormone, and *oxyphil cells*, whose contribution is still unknown. Having just one task to perform may sound like a fairly simple assignment, but there is more calcium in the body than any other mineral. The average adult body contains about 2½ pounds of calcium, and approximately 99% of it is stored in the bones.

The calcium level in the blood is regulated by the interaction of three products: parathyroid hormone, vitamin D, and calci-

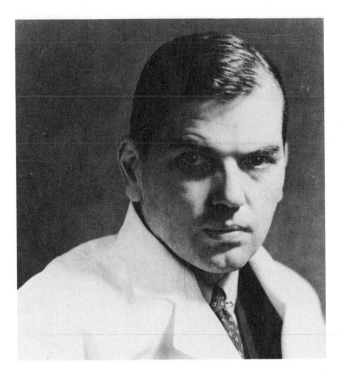

*The Boston physician
Fuller Albright*

tonin (the thyroid hormone discussed earlier in this chapter). They in turn affect three target tissues; bone, kidneys, and the gastrointestinal tract.

Action and Reaction

When the parathyroid receives signals that the level of calcium in the blood is too low, it releases the parathyroid hormone. This action immediately affects three bodily processes. First, the kidneys are sent instructions to reabsorb vitamin D, which allows for the release of the vitamin's active product, *metabolite*. This substance increases the amount of calcium the gastrointestinal tract can absorb. Thus, the body becomes more efficient in extracting and holding calcium from the food a person eats. Second, parathyroid hormone activates *osteoclasts*. These are cells that can actually break down bone tissue, extract the calcium, and return it to the blood. This also requires sufficient amounts of vitamin D metabolites for maximum effect. Finally, parathyroid hormone instructs the kidneys to reabsorb or save calcium that filters through them and return it to the circulatory system.

The control of calcium levels provides an example of both a negative and a positive feedback control mechanism. Once levels of circulating calcium begin to rise, signals are sent to the parathyroids to shut down production of parathyroid hormone. This is typical of negative feedback. At the same time, however, a rising level of serum calcium signals the thyroid to take action and boost secretion of calcitonin. As described in the section on the thyroid gland, calcitonin works to decrease calcium in the blood. It activates *osteoblasts*, which help form bone tissue from calcium, and it encourages the elimination of calcium from the body.

When the glands of the endocrine system are functioning properly, the body is able to balance its level of calcitonin and parathyroid hormone and keep blood calcium at normal levels. As with all living organs, however, the thyroid and parathyroids are subject to a variety of breakdowns.

Hypo- and Hyperparathyroidism

As with all the other hormones, the secretion of too much or too little parathyroid hormone upsets the body's ability to function properly. The right amount of circulating calcium is necessary if nerve cells are to remain in a resting state. If blood calcium levels drop too low, nerves will activate without an appropriate stimulus. This can result in twitching muscles, spasms, and even convulsions. These symptoms of hypoparathyroidism are known as *tetany*.

The most common cause of an underactive parathyroid is its accidental removal during the intended removal or surgical exploration of the thyroid gland. (If both the parathyroid's minute size and its attachment to the thyroid is taken into account, this will not seem as unlikely as it might to the uninformed patient.) Fortunately, hypoparathyroidism is readily treated with vitamin D and calcium, both of which can be taken orally.

Hyperparathyroidism is most common in people over 40; 188 out of every 200,000 women over the age of 60 are affected. (Men are affected less than half as often.) An adenoma on just one of the parathyroids is the cause in about 90% of these cases. Although nearly half of the people with hyperparathyroidism never show any symptoms, the excessive release of parathyroid hormone can prove harmful to bones, kidneys, and intestines. Calcium-depleted bones lose density and become weak. They are much more readily fractured or damaged. Excess quantities of calcium in the kidneys can encourage obstructions and kidney failure. In the gastrointestinal organs, hypercalcemia may cause constipation or nausea. Surgery is the most common treatment for patients suffering chronic symptoms of hyperparathyroidism.

•   •   •   •

CHAPTER 4

THE ADRENAL GLANDS

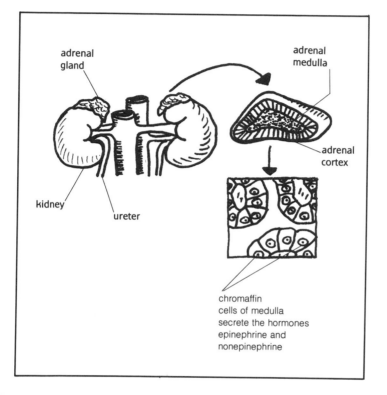

adrenal gland

adrenal medulla

adrenal cortex

kidney

ureter

chromaffin cells of medulla secrete the hormones epinephrine and nonepinephrine

The adrenal gland is essential to survival. Without it, humans would lose their life-saving ability to adapt to stress.

Latin scholars will know immediately where to look for the adrenal glands. For the rest of us, the translation should not be too difficult. In Latin, ad means "toward" or "near," and renes means "kidney." In this case, ad means very near. One adrenal gland perches atop each kidney like a triangular ski hat. Each gland is composed of two parts that produce their own distinct products and operate independently of each other. You could say that the adrenal is two glands in one.

The average adrenal gland weighs less than one-fourth of an ounce, or about five grams. It is less than two inches in length and about one inch wide. About 80% of the gland is composed of a yellowish outer section called the *cortex*. The inner portion is called the medulla. Like the thyroid, the *medulla* is saturated by blood vessels, which give it a deep red color.

THE ADRENAL CORTEX

Of all the glands discussed so far in this book, and of all that are to come, none is more crucial than the adrenal cortex. Without the ability to adapt to constant change, the human body would perish. And if not for the hormones of the adrenal cortex, even the slightest change or stress would prove lethal.

The pituitary controls the delicate operation of the adrenal cortex by regulating ACTH secretion. The adrenal cortex itself manufactures as many as 30 different hormones. These can then be divided into three types of hormones, all of which share the similar structure of the steroid. Each of these steroids derives from the same cholesterol origin. Although "healthy heart" advocates have been giving cholesterol bad press recently, its presence in reasonable amounts is actually crucial to the production of these cortex steroids, or *corticosteroids*.

The adrenal cortex is composed of three specialized layers, or zones. From the outermost to the deepest inner layer they are respectively called the *zona glomerulosa, zona fasciculata,* and *zona reticularis.* The following discussion of the adrenal cortex will be divided into a description of the function and structure of each of these zones.

Zone One: The Glomerulosa

Aldosterone is the primary hormone secreted in the outer layer, or zona glomerulosa, of the adrenal cortex. The level of aldosterone in the blood has a direct effect on the functioning of the kidneys. As aldosterone levels rise, the body retains salt and excretes potassium. The additional salt, or sodium, causes fluid retention; hypertension may result if excessive levels of aldosterone are maintained over a long period of time. Fortunately, the body has several fail-safe techniques to counteract this. When sodium levels become excessive, chemical signals are sent to the kidneys to stop them from reabsorbing the circulating sodium. Excesses are then excreted in the urine.

Zone Two: The Fasciculata

All it takes is a really bad case of poison oak, or an encounter with a medicine or food that causes huge red welts to appear on the skin, or a horrifying moment when the throat begins to close up and breathing becomes difficult, and one is likely to retain vivid memories of the healing power of cortisone. This miraculous drug is made from *cortisol*, the hormone produced in the zona fasciculata, or central section, of the adrenal cortex. An injection of this steroid can bring a severe allergic reaction under control literally in seconds. In pill form, cortisone is widely used to treat many serious illnesses, such as bronchial asthma, rheumatoid arthritis, and ulcerative colitis. As a cream, it heals a wide range of skin conditions.

Normally, the body secretes about 20 milligrams, or two-thirds of an ounce, of cortisol a day. This is nearly 200 hundred times the production of aldosterone. Cortisol regulates ACTH secretion, maintains blood pressure, regulates fluid levels, directs the metabolism of protein and glucose, increases or decreases body fat, and affects the immune system. Under extreme stress, the adrenals immediately begin pumping cortisol into the body. The output of cortisol can reach up to 20 times its normal production. This provides the body with emergency supplies of energy. Cortisol literally cannibalizes amino acids from muscles and fat from tissues. The metabolism goes into overdrive, and the immune system backs off. Stores of energy are readily at hand.

These transformations are very effective if one is combating a serious internal injury or facing a specific physical threat from the outside world. However, the day-to-day emotional stress of modern life can also cause an abnormally high secretion of cortisol. And if a person remains in a continual state of alert, serious stress-related disorders may develop. (More will be said about

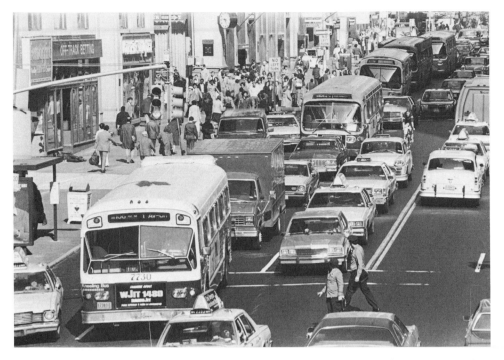

People who live in large urban centers often contend with overcrowded streets, traffic jams, and hectic schedules. Such constant stress can cause the adrenal cortex and medulla to produce a dangerous over-abundance of cortisol and adrenaline.

the repercussions of unremitting psychological stress in the discussion of the adrenal medulla.)

Excessively high levels of cortisol can also lead to a condition known as Cushing's syndrome. This is often the inadvertent consequence of treating an ailment with cortisol itself. Cushing's syndrome also frequently results from a malfunctioning pituitary that is putting out far too much ACTH. Yet another reason for the overproduction of cortisol is the growth of pituitary tumors, which may call for surgical removal.

Patients with Cushing's syndrome exhibit an array of visible symptoms. Obesity is common. Often the face gets so fat that it appears to be round. The trunk of the body also takes on weight, its excessive fat frequently forming what is commonly called a "buffalo hump." Bones become very weak, and disabling back problems are frequent. Abnormally high blood glucose and diabetes can result. Hypertension is frequent. Muscle weakness and a propensity to bruise are also common. From the severity of these reactions, it is obvious that medical professionals must monitor long-term cortisol treatments with extreme care.

It is also important that patients taking these medications be slowly weaned from them. During the course of treatment, the increase of cortisol alters several crucial bodily functions. The hypothalamus receives a signal causing it to shut down its production of ACTH. This in turn deactivates the adrenal cortex, whose production of hormones stop. Therefore, the dosage of cortisol must be gradually decreased to allow sufficient time for the reactivation of these hormones. If cortisol treatment is suddenly halted, cortisol levels may become dangerously low. This can lead to a greater risk of infection as well as to general weakness and weight loss. Until the adrenals kick in and begin producing hormones again, they cannot react, even to a minor crisis. A minor illness or injury might lead quite suddenly to an unexpected death.

Zone Three: The Reticularis

The innermost zone of the adrenal cortex, the *reticularis*, produces the sex hormones androgen and estrogen. The primary source for these hormones is not the adrenal glands but rather the gonads. The adrenals do play an important role, however, by providing men with some of the "female" hormone and women with some of the "male" hormone.

Although estrogen has little known effect in men, androgen's effect on women is more apparent. At puberty, it causes a variety of changes. Girls begin to grow pubic and underarm hair. Their voices may get somewhat deeper, and the first awakenings of sexual desire may begin. On the downside, androgen is also thought to be the culprit that encourages teenage acne.

ONE PROBLEM LEADS TO ANOTHER

In the rare event that the synthesis of cortisol steroids is blocked, the hypothalamus signals to the pituitary that there is a problem. The pituitary responds by secreting extra quantities of ACTH to stimulate cortisol production. However, since ACTH also con-

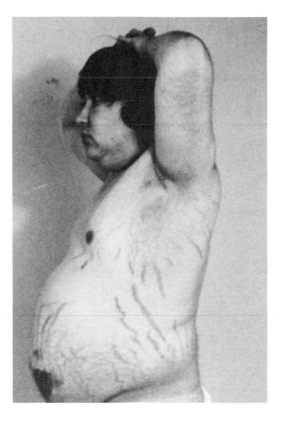

A sufferer of Cushing's syndrome. Symptoms of this condition, which can result from an overproduction of cortisol, are obesity, weakened bones, and a propensity to bruise.

trols the secretion of sex hormones from the adrenals, a high level of ACTH is likely to cause an overproduction of sex hormones. And the excessive amounts of androgen and estrogen pouring from the adrenals can cause a condition known as *virilization* to develop.

The results, if unchecked, can be quite dramatic. In the past, circus sideshows profited from this malady by exhibiting bearded ladies, along with dwarfs and giants, as freaks of nature. If the condition occurs when girls are quite young, they can even develop masculine genitals. Young males can also be affected. Babies and small boys can enter a premature puberty. Penis size increases, and bodily hair sprouts. As their sex organs are not yet mature, however, their testes will not produce hormones. As might be suspected, cortisol therapy is the most effective treatment for this condition.

THE MEDULLA

The inner section of the adrenal glands is known as the medulla. For those who have been wondering where adrenaline has been keeping itself, this is where it resides. The medulla secretes two hormones: *epinephrine*, commonly called adrenaline; and *norepinephrine*, better known as noradrenaline. Adrenaline is both the more potent and much more prevalent of the two, making up 80% of the medulla's hormones.

Nerve impulses excite the medulla to pump adrenaline and noradrenaline into the bloodstream. If you have ever been startled by a door slamming, very nearly run over by a truck, or followed down a dark street, you know exactly what a surge of these hormones feels like. (These are variations on the fight-or-flight response mentioned at the beginning of the book.) Your

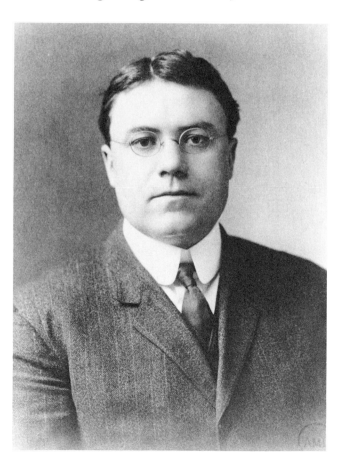

Dr. Walter Cannon

heart begins racing. Your breath comes faster. You are suddenly and intensely alert. Within seconds, your entire muscular system is capable of extraordinary feats. Your body has prepared you to either stand up to the emergency situation or physically remove yourself from it.

In 1931, Dr. Walter Cannon of Harvard University formulated the emergency theory of adrenaline secretion. While running experiments on a cat, he noticed that when the animal was calm, the blood circulating out of the adrenal gland was normal. When a dog was allowed into the laboratory, however, the cat's hormonal balance was significantly altered. Sudden secretions of adrenaline surged into its circulating blood.

The Stress Factor

Adrenaline and noradrenaline work in conjunction with the adrenal cortex hormone, cortisol. These are the main stress hormones. Under emergency conditions, they provide instant readiness for unusual physical demands as well as the energy needed to fulfill them. Although these hormonal reactions are extremely useful as a survival mechanism, problems can arise if this response is initiated too frequently.

Unfortunately, in modern society people are often subjected to an immoderate amount of daily stress, and the body may react to this stress as to an ongoing miniemergency. Although a deadline, a traffic jam, a missed appointment, or a final exam is rarely a life-and-death situation, many people become extremely agitated about such common occurrences.

Those people who live their entire life in a crisis mode fall into the category of what is called the "type A" personality. They always seem to be in a hurry and are continually under a lot of stress. They are generally impatient, preferring to be in complete control of a situation rather than delegating responsibility to someone else. They often say they work best under pressure.

The long-term consequences of such heightened hormonal activity can be very serious. The nearly constant release of stress hormones puts excessive demands on the body. The immune system can become depressed, leaving the body more susceptible to infections and disease. The cardiovascular system may be dam-

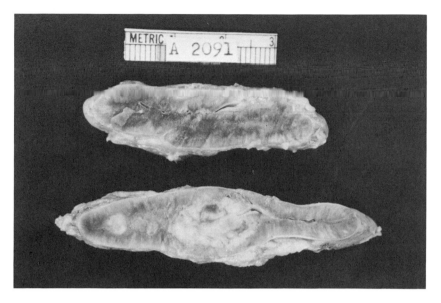

A healthy adrenal gland (top) and a tumorous one. Proper functioning of the adrenal gland is crucial to the fight-or-flight response.

aged by frequent and prolonged increases in blood pressure. This increases the risk of a heart attack or stroke. Current medical research shows that prolonged stress can also contribute to cancer, anorexia nervosa, suppressed growth, and diminished sex drive. The recognition and control of this behavior could save the life of a type A person.

There is an increasing body of research linking stress to loss of brain cells as well. Many scientists feel this may account for the rapid rise in Alzheimer's disease in modern society. This disease, which generally affects men and women who are 50 or older, is characterized by a progressive loss of mental ability, memory lapses, and extreme confusion.

Although the adrenal cortex and medulla work together to handle stress, there is an important difference between them. Unlike the adrenal cortex, the medulla is not a prerequisite to survival. The adrenal cortex responds primarily to pituitary stimulation, whereas the medulla responds to electrical messages sent directly from the nervous system. Fortunately, the nervous system can also do the work of adrenaline and noradrenaline in an emergency situation. At the same time as it excites the adrenal medulla, it telegraphs direct messages to the heart, lungs, and other vital organs. This provides an important fail-safe system. Even though the effects of these nerve impulses are 10 times weaker than those of hormonal messages, hypofunction of the adrenal medulla can be ruled out as a serious problem. In contrast, hyperfunction, which is most frequently caused by a tumor, must be treated. In such a case, either surgery or long-term drug therapy can prove effective.

•   •   •   •

CHAPTER 5

THE
PANCREAS

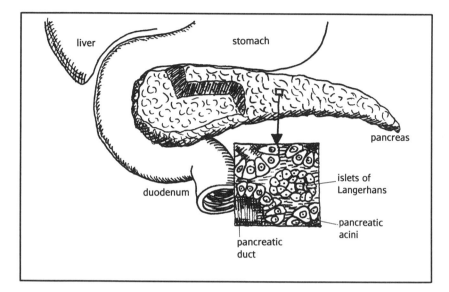

The pancreas produces a variety of hormones, including insulin, which helps remove glucose from the blood.

The pancreas is an elongated organ that generally measures six inches in length and lies sideways slightly below the stomach. As an exocrine organ, the pancreas produces enzymes that influence digestion. Our present concern with the pancreas, however, is with a tiny fraction of the organ that is composed of a cluster of hormone-producing cells referred to as the islets of Langerhans.

The hormone-producing cells of the pancreas are named for Paul Langerhans. It was Langerhans who in the late 1860s first

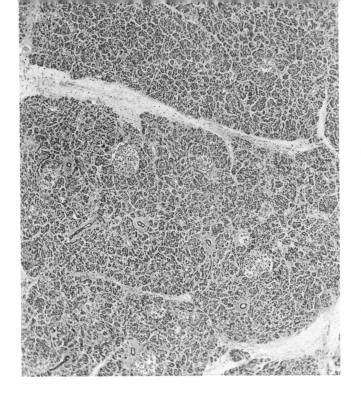

Islets of Langerhans
(× 50). About 1 million
of these tiny hormone-
producing cells occupy
less than 2% of
the pancreas.

described the existence of cells within the pancreas that were not connected to ducts. Later scientists discovered that these scattered cells actually operated as an endocrine gland. Estimates of the number of Langerhans' islets occupying a normal pancreas vary, but some go as high as 1 million. You can imagine how small they must be if all together they make up less than 2% of the entire pancreas.

Scientists have identified three types of cells within each of these miniscule islets. They are known as alpha, beta, and delta cells. Delta cells secrete somatostatin, but no one is quite sure what its purpose is. For now, it is enough to realize it exists. The beta cells, which comprise approximately 80% of the islets, manufacture and secrete *insulin*. This hormone helps remove glucose from the blood by binding to receptor cells and increasing its target tissue's ability to take up and use glucose. *Glucagon*, the hormone produced by the alpha cells, works in direct opposition to insulin—it increases blood sugar. Unlike many of the hormones presented in previous chapters, neither insulin nor glucagon is controlled by the pituitary gland. Both alpha and beta cells receive signals directly from the circulating blood and the nervous system. With a balance of insulin and glucagon secretions, the body is able to constantly adjust its level of circulating glucose.

BREAKING DOWN AND BUILDING UP

Meeting the daily needs of every organ in the body requires an enormous amount of energy. Even when a person is sleeping or sitting perfectly still, billions of cells continue to function, and they all have to be fed. To add to the complexity, different organs have different requirements. The brain demands a constant diet of pure glucose and is the largest consumer of glucose in the entire body. Whether you are puzzling through a homework assignment in advanced trigonometry or playing with your cat, your brain's appetite stays at nearly the exact same level. If supplies of blood sugar fall too low, the brain will stop functioning at full capacity almost immediately. In comparison, muscles like

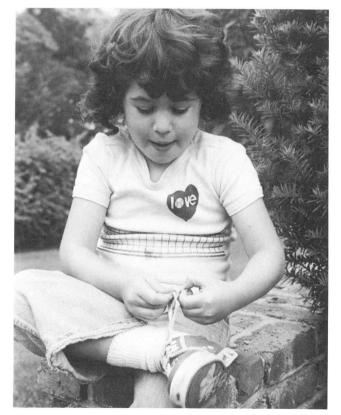

The brain requires the same amount of glucose for simple tasks—such as tying a shoelace—as it does for complex ones.

a mixture of glucose, fat, and protein. The heart thrives on mostly fat, some glucose, and just a dash of protein.

Much of the body's blood sugar is derived from carbohydrates. After a meal, glucose levels in the blood rise. This triggers the release of insulin from the pancreas. The insulin circulates through the body and attaches itself to receptors on the appropriate cells. Muscle cells are particularly well supplied with insulin receptors. Once the insulin is in place, it allows glucose to enter the cell, where it is used as energy. When levels of insulin are high, glucose that is not metabolized or used right away is turned into *glycogen* and stored in the liver. Some is also converted into fat and stored in the adipose, or "fatty," tissues. These fat cells are known as *triglycerides*. Excess carbohydrate molecules are used in this conversion. Adipose tissue insulates the body from cold and heat and serves as a convenient reserve bank for energy. Thus, insulin lowers blood sugar levels both by getting glucose into the cells that need it and by converting it into products for storage.

Glucagon, the hormone produced by the alpha cells, has the reverse function. It increases the amount of glucose in circulation. When sugar levels fall too low, alpha cells are stimulated. Glucagon production rises, and glycogen stored in the liver is converted back into glucose. The liver releases the glucose into the blood, and blood sugar increases. Amino acids can also be converted into glucose if necessary. Glucagon can affect its secretion, as well as that of adrenaline and cortisol from the adrenal gland and growth hormone from the pituitary.

DIABETES

When insulin supplies are deficient, or when the body is unable to use supplies of insulin, blood sugar levels rise to dangerous levels. This condition is known as hyperglycemia, and recognition of its symptoms led to identification and, eventually, to treatment of the disease called diabetes mellitus.

This disease has been known for several thousand years, and the original meaning of its name accurately describes its most prevalent, observable symptoms. The ancient Greeks referred to it as *diabetes*, meaning "siphon," and in the late 17th century the Latin word *mellitus*, meaning "honey-sweet," was added. The siphoning, or excretion, of vast quantities of urine containing extremely high concentrations of sugar is an early sign of diabetes mellitus.

Excessive amounts of sugar in the blood reduce the kidneys' ability to absorb water. This results in *polyuria*, a drastic increase in urination. In turn, this creates *polydipsia*, a desperate thirst. At the same time, although the sugar level is high, it is not reaching the cells that need it. The body is starving for energy, and *polyphagia*, or excessive eating, is common. Unable to use glucose—its main source of energy—the body will begin using stores of protein as an alternative fuel. This causes protein deficiencies. As a result, healing and infection fighting become more difficult.

When there is a lack of insulin, or if insulin is not able to perform, the liver begins to break down reserve stores of fat. This causes weight loss and also releases an acidic product called *ketones*. Ketones give the breath a peculiar odor that can be mistaken for alcohol. In some unfortunate cases, diabetics have gone into a coma and died because bystanders assumed they were drunk rather than in need of immediate medical attention. Most doctors encourage their diabetic patients to wear medical alert bracelets. These have saved hundreds of thousands of lives.

Medical alert bracelets have saved the life of many thousands of diabetics. If the diabetic should fall into a coma, such bracelets inform bystanders that medical attention is necessary.

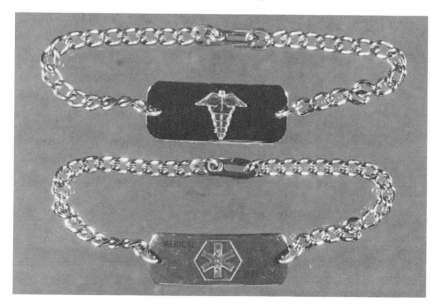

In the United States alone there are currently over 4 million diabetics; over 100,000 new cases of diabetes mellitus are diagnosed each year. And the number is rising. Diabetes is the third leading cause of death in the United States, behind only heart disease and cancer. Having diabetes doubles the chance of having a fatal heart attack or stroke. It causes at least 20% of all kidney failures, and it is the leading cause of blindness in adults.

Unfortunately, there is no cure for diabetes. There are, however, many excellent treatments currently available that allow most diabetic patients to lead a fairly normal life. In many cases, effective therapy depends directly on the patients' ability to take an active interest in monitoring and treating themselves.

Early detection of diabetes is now often possible. A laboratory test called a glucose tolerance test (GTT) is used to identify the prediabetic, and recent advances in at-home blood tests now offer easy, accurate, and safe testing of glucose levels. Susceptibility to diabetes mellitus increases in adults over the age of 45, and after the age of 30 it is more commonly found in women than in men. Obese people are more likely to get diabetes than are people of normal weight. Diabetes also tends to be genetically transmitted, so those whose families have a history of diabetes should be exceptionally aware that its early diagnosis can mean the difference between life and death.

Type I and Type II Diabetes

Type I diabetes mellitus goes by at least two other names. It was originally called *juvenile-onset* diabetes, because it is commonly seen in people under the age of 20. It is also referred to as *insulin-dependent* diabetes. Type I diabetics do not produce sufficient insulin. In many cases, the cause is genetic. In others, it is brought on by viruses that destroy the beta cells of the pancreas. It can also be caused by a haywire immune reaction in which the body mistakenly creates antibodies that kill its own beta cells. Onset of the disease is generally rapid, and patients must receive replacement insulin daily. Generally, patients or their parents learn how to test blood glucose levels and how to administer the daily injections.

Type II diabetes mellitus is characterized by the inability of the body to use insulin. This form of diabetes, also known as

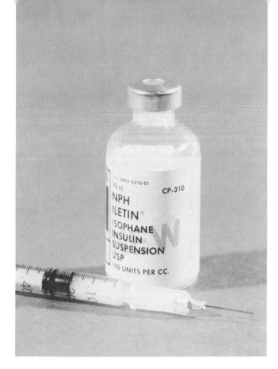

Daily injections of insulin have proved to be a successful form of treatment for diabetes mellitus. In most cases, patients can lead a normal, healthy life.

adult-onset or *non-insulin-dependent* diabetes, is much more common than type I. Type II accounts for 80% of all cases. This form of diabetes is also very frequently caused by genetic factors.

Regardless of whether insulin production is low, high, or normal, the body cannot use it effectively. The dysfunction can occur at any of several stages. The attachment of the insulin to the cell may not be effective. Insulin receptors may be lacking. The ability of insulin to attract glucose may be impeded. The hormone may fail to effectively transport the glucose into the target cell.

Obesity has been proven to interfere significantly with insulin receptors. Not surprisingly, many type II diabetics are obese. If they are able to get their weight back to normal, their receptors can work again. Some sufferers of type II diabetes find it necessary to take insulin or oral medication. For the most part, however, the treatment of type II diabetics focuses on diet and exercise.

HYPOGLYCEMIA

If you have ever tried a high-protein, low-cholesterol diet, you may have experienced some of the symptoms of mild hypoglycemia. Perhaps you felt light-headed or weak. Your vision may have been blurry, and you may have had trouble concentrating. You might have even experienced some trembling or heart palpitations. And, needless to say, you probably felt like you were starving. In some respects, you were. Your body was starving for sugar. Hypoglycemia is a condition that results when blood sugar levels fall too low. This is why it is very important for anyone who wants to diet to do so under proper medical supervision. Some people experience mild hypoglycemia if they skip a meal or wait too long to eat. For them and for the dieter, an intake of sugar or carbohydrates will provide immediate relief. For the diabetic, however, it can be more complicated.

Hypoglycemia is a common complication of insulin therapy, for too much of this substance depletes blood sugar levels rapidly. Type I and type II diabetics must be able to recognize the onset of hypoglycemia and take action instantly. If they delay, serious consequences can result. Usually drinking some orange juice or eating a candy bar will sufficiently restore glucose levels. If action is postponed, however, severe hypoglycemia can develop. The person can fall into a coma or suffer serious brain damage. Oral medications do exist for patients who cannot readily control hypoglycemia through diet.

Scientists are making rapid progress in the treatment of diabetes. They are developing insulin pumps that will deliver a continual flow of insulin to the bloodstream. This will help to maintain proper glucose levels even while the patient sleeps. Islet cell transplants and pancreas transplant operations are also in the experimental stage. If successful, they would offer a long-term solution to many thousands of people with insufficient insulin production.

•   •   •   •

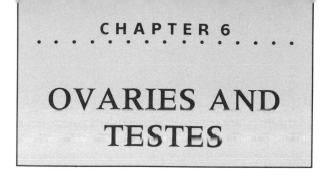

CHAPTER 6

OVARIES AND TESTES

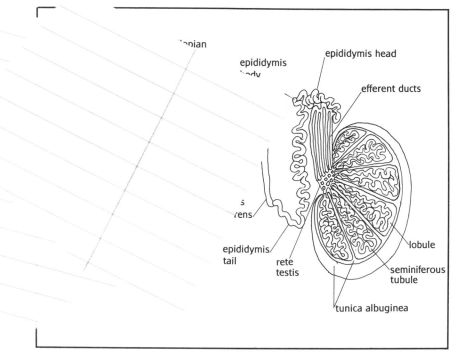

epididymis body

epididymis head

efferent ducts

'anian

rens

epididymis tail

rete testis

lobule

seminiferous tubule

tunica albuginea

An ovary and testis

L ike the other endocrine glands, which usually go unnoticed unless they malfunction, the testes in men and the ovaries in women play a crucial role. Their pervasive influence is particularly evident during the teenage years, when sex hormones surge and sexual maturation takes place. At no other time, except perhaps in the first few years of life (and most of us do not remember much of that), do our bodies undergo such dramatic and rapid changes. Sex hormones affect much more than physical appearance, and their control extends even beyond the physiological processes of sexual maturation and reproduction. They also hold sway over emotions and attitudes by opening up a whole spectrum of desire.

IN THE BEGINNING

Sexual development begins at the instant of conception. The fertilized egg carries within it every piece of genetic information it will ever need to produce every type of cell for a lifetime. Thus, from the very beginning, it is determined whether an embryo will mature into a male or female. Sex organs begin to show up very early in fetal development. Testicles begin to emerge in about the seventh week, and ovaries start to form in the 16th week. Sex hormone levels in the developing fetus are high. These hormones directly influence the fetal development of the sex glands.

Some medical experts believe that these early hormones affect the developing brain and contribute to behavioral differences between men and women. There are others, though, experts or not, who argue vehemently against this. These people believe that social factors, not biological ones, are solely responsible for the differences between how men and women act.

Once a baby is born, its sex hormone production drastically reduces. No one is sure what function sex hormones serve in children. Although the testes and ovaries of children are capable of manufacturing and secreting hormones, the pituitary gland has not yet provided the activating signals.

GONADS AND OVARIES

The male gonads, or testes, have a unique location. They lie suspended between the thighs in a sac called the *scrotum*. The testes are situated outside the body because they need a lower temperature to produce viable sperm. These two egg-shaped organs are about two inches long and together weigh less than an ounce. They have two main components. The *seminiferous tubules* are long, narrow, curling tubes in which sperm cells are formed. These tubes are tightly packed into the testes and com-

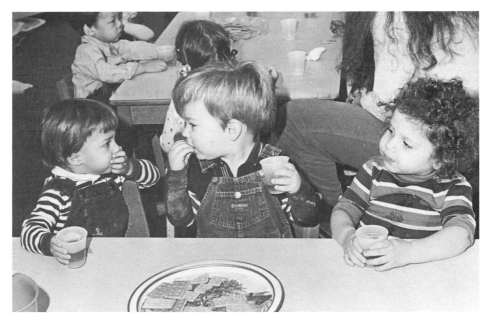

Because the pituitary gland does not activate its sexual hormones until adolescence, it is sometimes difficult to distinguish prepubescent girls from boys.

pose about 95% of the glands. The little spaces between the tubes hold *Leydig's cells*. These cells produce nearly all of the androgens, including *testosterone*, the major androgen hormone secreted by the testes.

Ovaries are the female gonads. One sits on each side of the uterus and is attached to it by ligaments. They are oval-shaped and measure about an inch and a half in length. Ovaries vary in weight in different stages of a female's life but weigh the most during the years that she is fertile. The ovaries produce the hormones *estrogen, progesterone*, and *relaxin*. At birth, the ovaries of a female already contain all of the egg-forming cells, or follicles, she will ever produce. It is thought that females begin with a supply of 2 million of these follicles. Only one is used each month in the development of a mature egg.

Like the hormones of the adrenal cortex, hormones of the sex glands are steroids. Although they share a similar carbohydrate origin, they are crucially different in final form and function. Each gland contains particular enzymes that account for the

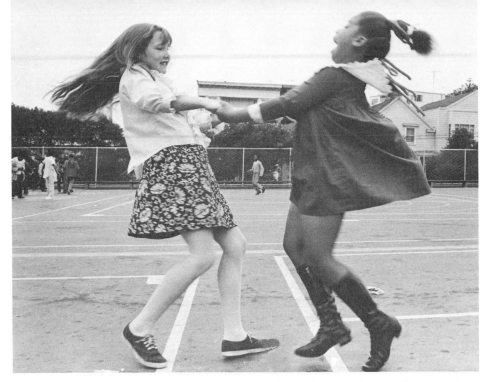

The characteristics distinguishing children from adults are the same for all people. But each individual goes through these changes at his or her own pace.

synthesis of specific steroids. The manufacture and secretion of the gonads is under the control of the hypothalamus and the pituitary.

PUBERTY

Have you ever complimented a mother on her darling baby girl only to learn it was a boy? Or perhaps you called her son a girl. Do not worry; it happens to all of us. Aside from genitals, physical differences in the bodies and faces of young boys and girls are not all that different. In fact, if it were not for hairstyles and outfits, the confusion would probably continue until puberty.

As was mentioned earlier, not everyone begins puberty at the same age. In the United States, girls begin puberty somewhere between the ages of 8 and 14. Boys start about two years later than girls, usually in their early teens. There seems to be neither a set pattern nor a standard pace at which the many physical changes of puberty occur.

One boy may shoot up to a height of 5 feet 7 inches in his early teens, whereas his friend hardly grows at all until suddenly at age 17, when he spurts up to become a 6-foot man. One boy will grow a heavy beard early on, and another will not need to shave until he is in college. In the same way, one girl may begin menstruating when she is 10 years old, whereas another will not start until she is 16; yet a third girl will develop breasts in grade school, causing her best friend to worry about her own as-yet undeveloped ones. Each child has his or her own individual way of transforming into a man or woman.

It takes approximately seven years to pass from childhood into adulthood. Although puberty seems to last forever for those who are going through it, enormous bodily changes occur in a remarkably brief span of time. Puberty is characterized by a rapid increase in growth, the development of secondary sex characteristics, and the maturation of reproductive organs.

At no other time does such rapid growth occur, aside from the earliest infant years. The pituitary is stimulated to increase the production of growth hormone. Once this occurs, most children grow about 25% taller in just 4 years. No wonder many teenagers feel suddenly gawky and awkward. Their bodies have become incredible growing machines.

Secondary Sex Characteristics

In addition, the pituitary, under the direction of the hypothalamus, releases hormones that strike up activity in the gonads. The production and release of sex hormones, which were suppressed during childhood, now surge. Physical changes start occurring from head to toe. This is often both a very exciting and a very confusing time. Suddenly, *secondary sex characteristics* become apparent. These are physical attributes that separate men from women but are not directly involved in reproduction.

In girls, breast development tends to be the first sign. Generally, the nipples and the areolae, the dark areas that surround them, begin to grow. This is followed by the arrival of soft pubic hair and underarm hair. Weight increases as hips and thighs become more rounded. As development progresses, breasts increase in size, and pubic hair becomes darker and coarser.

In boys, the first sign of the onset of puberty is most often an increase in the size of the testicles. This is caused by an enlargement of the seminiferous tubules. Soon after, the penis also begins to enlarge. Facial hair, pubic hair, and underarm hair begin to sprout. The larynx, or voice box, grows larger, causing the voice to deepen. This change in the voice can happen gradually or very suddenly. The shoulders and chest enlarge, muscles develop, and weight increases.

TESTOSTERONE

Testosterone has a tremendous influence on a boy's transformation into a man. This hormone is responsible for both the growth and differentiation of the male genitals. It also stimulates the growth of bodily hair and the production of sperm. (Testosterone is also present in women, but in much smaller amounts.) And the list goes on. The level of a man's testosterone plays an essential role in the texture of his skin and hair, the speed at which he metabolizes food, how deep a voice he will have, whether he will lose his hair or not, and even how massive his muscles and bones will become.

The Potential for Abuse

It is this tissue-building, or anabolic, effect of testosterone that has spurred an illegal market in steroids. If you watched the

The world-renowned Vienna Boys Choir has been in existence for close to 500 years. Its singing is consistently clear and high-pitched because each member must leave the choir as soon as his voice deepens.

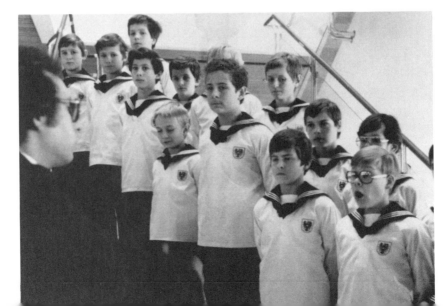

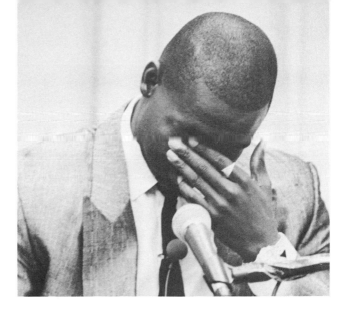

television coverage of the 1988 Summer Olympics in Seoul, South Korea, you are sure to remember Ben Johnson's incredible performance. Running the 100-meter race, Johnson got off to a blazing start and left the competition far behind. He ran the race in 9.79 seconds, setting a new world record and winning a gold medal.

Three days after the race, however, the Olympic Committee stripped Johnson of the prize. Blood tests showed that the Canadian runner had been taking anabolic steroids. These are synthetic hormones that were developed to duplicate the effects of testosterone.

Although medical experts disagree as to whether steroids can improve athletic ability, they all agree that taking an abnormal amount of them can have harmful effects that may last a lifetime. In large quantities, over a long period of time, anabolic steroids can be very dangerous. In young men, they can speed up the maturation process. This can result in stunted growth or early baldness. Young girls who take steroids run the risk of developing masculine traits that will not disappear, even when they stop taking the drugs.

As it does with many other hormones, a negative feedback system regulates the secretion of testosterone to prevent its overproduction or underproduction. Athletes taking large doses of steroids are seriously challenging their bodies' ability to maintain a proper balance of testosterone. This can eventually lead to heart disease or kidney and liver damage and may even increase the risk of liver cancer. When massive amounts of anabolic steroids are present in the body, the pituitary may shut down testosterone production. In the male, this can cause the testes to shrink and breasts to develop.

Testosterone and Sexuality

Testosterone is responsible for igniting sexual desire in both men and women. So far, estrogen and progesterone, although very important to sexual reproduction, have not shown any relationship to desire. Men who have lost interest in sex frequently show an abnormally low testosterone level. Injections of this hormone can restore their sex drive. This works for both men and women. Generally though, testosterone levels remain relatively constant throughout a man's life from puberty until about age 40. After that, the levels gradually decline over the next 40 years until the sex drive and fertility are decreased by about 20%.

Although hormonal levels greatly influence the sexual behavior of both men and women, any discussion of human sexuality must consider not only hormonal influences but also the important part thoughts and feelings play concerning one's sexual drive. Moreover, no matter how much work is done studying the factors that determine a person's sex drive, human sexuality remains, to a degree, a mysterious and fluctuating aspect of life.

Taking steroids to increase physical ability exposes the athlete to tremendous health risks further down the line.

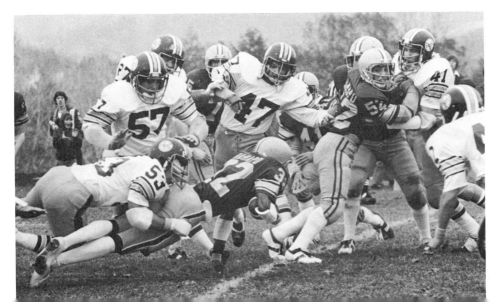

THE REPRODUCTIVE CYCLE

Unlike testosterone, which is controlled by a negative feedback system, the release of estrogen and progesterone is cyclical. One period, known as the menstrual cycle, normally extends over 28 days. In pubescent girls, menstruation may begin months or even years before regular ovulation begins. Adolescent girls may begin by producing sufficient hormones to build up and shed the uterine lining each month but not enough to produce a mature egg.

Once sexual maturation is complete, however, the menstrual cycle follows a specific pattern, beginning with the release of FSH from the pituitary. This stimulates the development of an egg in one of the ovaries. As the egg grows, the follicle secretes estrogen. This prevents the pituitary from releasing additional FSH, so no other eggs begin to mature. Estrogen also causes the uterus to prepare to receive a fertilized egg by building up a lining. As estrogen levels rise, the pituitary secretes LH, which in turn causes the ovary to release the egg into the oviduct. Once the egg is on its own, the leftover body that held the egg—the corpus luteum—begins producing progesterone. This hormone stops the pituitary from releasing either FSH or LH.

If the egg is not fertilized, the corpus luteum gives up and stops producing progesterone. This will generally happen a couple of days after the egg is released. As the level of progesterone declines, the thick lining of the uterus breaks up and causes the bleeding known as menstrual flow. At the same time, the pituitary, which is no longer suppressed, begins to produce FSH again. This starts the cycle once more.

The surges and falls in hormonal levels during the course of a menstrual cycle affect women in many different ways. The sudden rise of progesterone can cause women to feel particularly tense, depressed, or nervous. Many women also retain fluids and feel irritable and bloated several days before their period begins. In recent years, the term *premenstrual syndrome (PMS)* has been created to cover any or all of these symptoms. For most women, PMS is only an occasional or mild event. More than once, though, an extreme case of PMS has been used as a defense during the trial of a woman accused of murder. It is obviously important that women should contact their doctor if they suffer violent mood swings caused by alterations in hormone levels.

Controlling the Cycle

If the delicate hormonal balance that controls the woman's menstrual cycle is altered, conception can be very difficult, if not impossible. This is the basis upon which birth control pills work. Most of these contain a combination of estrogen and progesterone. They raise the level of hormones in the blood. The body treats this as a pregnancy and instructs the pituitary to shut off production of FSH and LH. This prevents the development and release of a mature egg. When the pills are discontinued for a few days each month, menstruation begins. Women who go off birth control pills are often surprised that they may skip their period for many months. Their body has become so accustomed to the excessively high hormone levels that their feedback system no longer works. It can take as long as half a year for the signals to return to normal.

Many women (and men) wonder why a birth control pill for males has not yet been developed. It may be, but progress is very slow. For women, only one event a month has to be controlled—the production and delivery of a mature egg. For men, who can produce more than a million sperm a day, the development of a birth control pill becomes far more complex.

Hormones and Pregnancy

When a woman becomes pregnant, her body begins producing and secreting more sex hormones than at any other time in her life. Cells of the embryo release a hormone that keeps the corpus luteum intact for the first three months. The corpus luteum enlarges and produces greater and greater amounts of both progesterone and estrogen. The progesterone helps the embryo receive nourishment from the uterus and prevents uterine contractions. It also helps prepare the breasts to produce milk. The estrogen causes the uterus and breasts to enlarge. By the end of the third month, the corpus luteum degenerates, and the placenta becomes an endocrine gland, supplying the fetus with the necessary quantities of estrogen and progesterone for its ongoing development.

By the end of the ninth month, the level of estrogen is so high that it counters the effect of progesterone on the uterus. At this point the body is preparing for labor. Contractions will be encouraged rather than prevented. Once labor begins, the mother's hypothalamus stimulates the posterior pituitary to release oxytocin. This hormone causes uterine contractions. At the same time, the mother's ovaries secrete *relaxin*. This hormone helps to dilate the cervix and the birth canal in preparation for the baby's delivery.

Infertility

Ten to fifteen percent of all couples are unable to conceive. This is often caused by a hormonal problem. Deficient sperm production or delivery accounts for 40% of the cases. A medical evaluation will usually determine where the problems stem from. The pituitary, ovaries, testes, and adrenal and thyroid glands should all be examined and their hormonal production tested in evaluating fertility problems.

MENOPAUSE

Although it may seem that the female body produces an enormous quantity of hormones throughout life, the opposite is true. Women produce no more than a teaspoonful of estrogen, for example, from the time puberty begins through the end of their reproductive years. The ending of fertility, like the beginning, is a process than can take several years. Most women experience it in three stages.

During the first stage, known as *premenopause*, the ovaries begin to produce fewer hormones. Menstrual flow often changes. For some women it lessens, while for others it becomes heavier. During *menopause*, the second stage, women stop having periods. Ovarian function has ceased or is very minimal. By the time a woman has gone through one year without having a period, she is said to be in stage three, or *postmenopause*.

Some women begin stage one in their forties, whereas others continue to have periods through their fifties. It is very unusual, however, for a woman to enter her sixties without having gone through all three stages.

Many women go through the process without experiencing any discomforting physical symptoms. For those who do, *hot flashes* are the most common source of complaints. These are very sudden and temporary rushes of heat that begin in the chest and spread upward. No one is quite sure what causes hot flashes, but they are known to originate in the hypothalamus. Another problem is painful intercourse. When estrogen secretion is curtailed, the tissue lining in the vagina thins, and vaginal secretions lessen. Fortunately, there are many creams available to alleviate this problem. In addition, estrogen replacement therapy in combination with progesterone is now being administered to many women. Test results to date show this combination to be an effective and safe treatment for many of the symptoms of menopause and postmenopause. There is no proven psychological advantage to hormone replacement therapy, aside from women's improved mental outlook when hot flashes have been eliminated and vaginal atrophy prevented. Physicians are therefore reluctant to prescribe hormone therapy for the depression that may accompany menopause. Relaxation techniques, counseling, or antidepressant drugs are much more commonly used.

•   •   •   •

CHAPTER 7

THE THYMUS AND PINEAL GLANDS

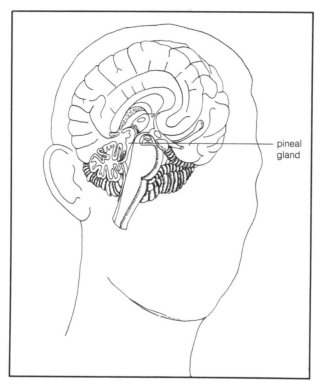

The pineal gland may be the remnant of a third eye still found in some lower animals.

The thymus could be called the incredible shrinking gland. Composed of two lobes held together by connective tissue, the thymus lies in the chest, behind the breastbone and above the heart. It is quite large in the newborn infant and continues to grow throughout childhood. It is at its heaviest just before puberty, weighing in at nearly an ounce and a half. From puberty on, however, it begins to shrink. The thymus is so small in adults that it is difficult to find during dissection.

FIGHTING FOREIGN INVADERS

Despite its tiny size, the thymus plays a crucial role in keeping the body in good health. Without it, the immune system could not function properly, and the body's ability to fight infection would be seriously impaired. When a bacteria, virus, or other foreign substance enters, the body must be able to recognize the invader immediately. The immune system has the amazing ability to distinguish cells that belong to the body (self cells) from invading (nonself) cells. Once recognition occurs, the immune system must then destroy these invaders before they multiply and take over. The cells comprising the forces of the immune system are called white blood cells.

These cells engulf foreign invaders, broadcast signals of the invasion, and call in reinforcements. The thymus plays a crucial role in the attack by producing a type of white cell known as the *T lymphocyte*, or T cell.

Millions of T cells are constantly circulating in the body, ever alert to rally in case of attack. From the time of birth every person has a wide variety of T cells. They help the immune system to combat not only known diseases, such as measles, but also the thousands of new germs that develop each year. T cells are activated through receptors on their cell walls. As they circulate, they come into contact with other white cells that have trapped invading cells.

The T cells respond in several ways. They immediately begin to divide and multiply in a maneuver known as cloning. Four types of T cells result: killer T cells that attack and destroy target cells; memory T cells that launch an immediate attack if the same invader shows up again; helper T cells that call in reinforcements; and suppressor T cells that call off the troops once the battle is under control.

Another class of white cells enter the fray when the helper T cells signal them. These are known as *B lymphocytes*, or B cells. Some activated B cells become plasma cells. These manufacture all of the antibodies the body produces to fight infection and disease. Antibodies seek out and coat foreign cells, making them easy targets for the many varieties of killer cells in circulation.

The separation of T cells into four categories and the activation of B cells are largely under the control of hormones manufactured in the thymus. To date, researchers have identified four different products: *thymosin, thymic humoral factor (THF), thymic factor (TF)*, and *thymopoietin*. There is still much to be learned about these hormones.

AIDS and the Immune System

Acquired immune deficiency syndrome (AIDS) is an acquired defect of the immune system that was officially recognized as an epidemic disease by the Centers for Disease Control in 1981. The AIDS virus can be passed from one person to another only through the exchange of bodily fluids, mainly blood or semen. Experts estimate that by the end of 1992, there will be as many as 365,000 people in the United States who have been diagnosed as having AIDS. Unless scientists make rapid progress in fighting

The thymus is quite large in an infant and continues to grow throughout childhood. It reaches its maximum weight at puberty, then shrinks drastically, and is barely discernible in full-grown adults.

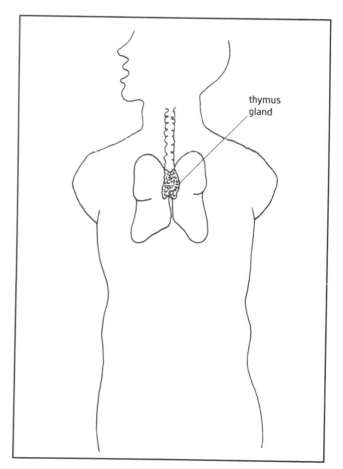

thymus gland

this disease, 263,000 of these people are expected to die. AIDS devastates the cells of the immune system, particularly T cells. It not only destroys cells but can also inactivate healthy cells from functioning properly.

Researchers are doing experiments on AIDS patients involving thymosin. They are testing to see if the hormone can help repair a damaged immune system. Noting that administering thymosin helped to reverse immune deficiencies in children born without thymus glands or with malfunctioning organs, they hope that boosting supplies of thymosin will increase the production and action of T cells and B cells in people with AIDS.

THE PINEAL GLAND

The tiny, deeply buried pineal gland has mystified researchers for centuries. René Descartes, one of the great thinkers of the 17th century, credited the pineal gland with being "the seat of the rational soul." Almost all fish, birds, reptiles, and mammals have pineal glands. This seems to have been the case for a very long time. Paleontologists, who study ancient fossils, have found evidence of pineal glands that goes back 500 million years. Although its exact function remains an enigma, the longevity of the pineal body alone indicates that it is clearly of some importance to human survival.

Still, a few things are known with certainty about this gland. The human variety is generally less than one-quarter of an inch long and weighs a fraction of a gram. It is cone shaped, or more exactly, pinecone shaped, which is how it got its name. The pineal resides close to the very center of the brain. At about the time of puberty, it begins to calcify. This produces calcium deposits known as *brain sand*. Do not worry, though; apparently, this partial calcification has nothing to do with the effective functioning of the brain.

The pineal gland is thought to be the only gland producing the hormone *melatonin*. In humans, melatonin is secreted throughout the night, and its secretion seems to be directly related to the absence of light. During the day, light enters the eyes. It sends signals through the optic nerve to the spinal cord. These signals are then carried by nerve impulses to the pineal gland. As long as these signals are received, melatonin production is shut down. During the day, the gland prepares for the evening's work by synthesizing amino acids into serotonin. Serotonin converts to melatonin under cover of night.

Melatonin was first discovered in 1958 by researchers at the Yale University School of Medicine. Their work, like much of the work on the pineal gland, was based on research with animals. It appears that melatonin levels directly control the breeding habits of most species. Species with a long gestation period, such as deer and bears, generally conceive in the fall and give birth in the spring. Animals with short gestation periods, such as rabbits and birds, reproduce in the spring and summer. This assures that newborns are given the best possible chance for survival. During the dark, harsh winter, melatonin production is up, and sexual activity is down.

AIDS virus attacking cell (× 150,000). By destroying cells of the immune system, the virus leaves the body vulnerable to a host of diseases.

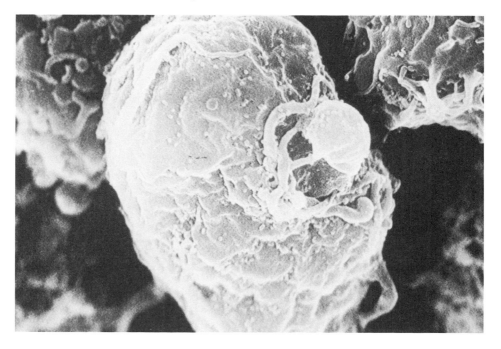

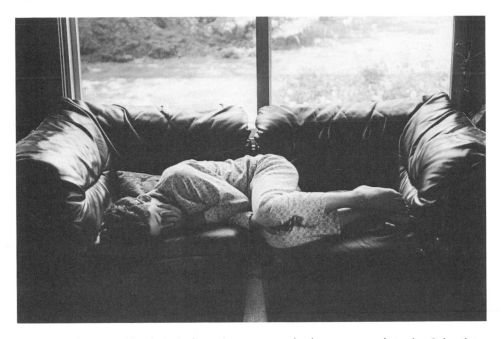

The pineal body is believed to secrete the hormone melatonin. Scientists believe that the level of melatonin rises when there is an absence of light, and this may be a reason many people are more tired and depressed during the winter months.

Seasonal Affective Disorder

In humans, rising levels of melatonin correlate with increased sleepiness, a craving for carbohydrates, and an inability to concentrate. People who live in climates that have long, dark winters often experience a seasonal depression. Perhaps you have had a case of the "winter blues." If you generally feel depressed, lethargic, withdrawn, and tend to gain weight in the winter, you may qualify as a victim of *SAD*, or *seasonal affective disorder*.

This newly identified mental health disorder is thought to affect over 25 million people in the United States alone. Most cases occur in the Northeast, the Great Lakes area, and in the states of Washington and Alaska. In some cases, symptoms can become extremely severe. People are unable to cope with even the slightest problems and can barely stay awake at all during the day.

Generally, victims of SAD feel better when spring arrives, and a vacation to a sunnier climate may help to relieve symptoms.

In addition, researchers have begun to experiment with light therapy. It has been found that exposing SAD patients to very bright lights for a few hours a day seems to cure their depression and craving for carbohydrates. Results often occur within a matter of two or three days. The level of light must be at least 10 times as bright as that of a normally brightly lit room.

Until recently, these high intensity light treatments were available only in research settings. However, Dr. George Brainard, a neurologist, and Dan Benson, a biomedical engineer, have invented a very special hat that may help to alleviate some of the symptoms of SAD victims. Under its brim are two six-inch lights that span the wearer's forehead. The lights are powered by a small, portable battery pack. Patients can go through their morning routines while receiving "light hat" treatments—it only takes

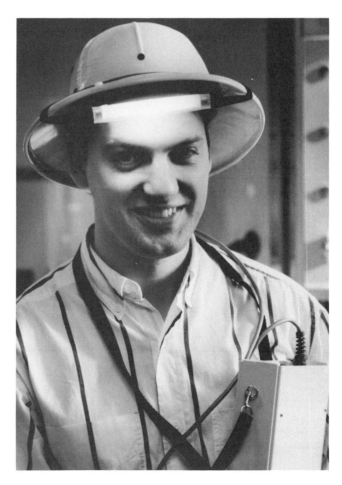

A sufferer of seasonal affective disorder wears a "light hat," which is thought to relieve symptoms of the condition, possibly because it suppresses melatonin secretion.

an hour or two a day. To date, Brainard and Benson report complete relief of all symptoms in 85% of their cases.

None of the researchers working with light treatments is absolutely certain why this therapy works. The common consensus, however, is that it suppresses melatonin secretion. Experts are also unsure about what effect, if any, melatonin has on human sexual activity. Many feel that high melatonin levels suppress gonadal development in young children. As melatonin levels fall prior to puberty, signals travel to the hypothalamus to activate the pituitary to stimulate the gonads. This connection between melatonin and sexual development is only a conjecture, though— one of the many mysteries of the pineal gland yet to be solved.

•   •   •   •

CHAPTER 8

WHAT THE FUTURE MAY BRING

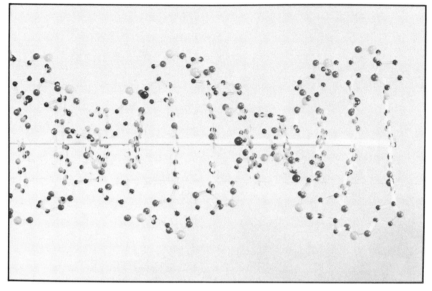

Model of DNA structure

Charles Edouard Brown-Séquard, a professor and investigator of medicine at the Collège de France, was one of the prominent figures in the study of endocrinology. Brown-Séquard taught that the adrenals, thyroid, pancreas, liver, spleen, and kidneys had secretions (later called hormones) that entered the bloodstream and could be used in treatment. In 1889, at the age of 72, he sought to prove his theory that injections of extracts from the testes would reverse the aging process. To that end, he

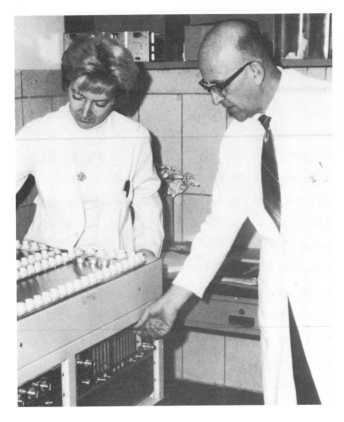

Medical technologists use a gamma counter to measure hormone concentrations in the blood and pituitary. This technique, developed in the late 1960s, is called radioimmunoassay.

injected himself with fluid he had extracted from a dog's testes. Although he claimed to feel instantly rejuvenated in both mind and body, his colleagues were unconvinced. And their rigorous tests showed that Brown-Séquard's enthusiasm had its source in his senility, rather than in the results of his experiment.

One hundred years later, scientists suspect that Professor Brown-Séquard may have shown considerably more insight than his detractors credited him with. Although scientists are far from reversing the aging process, hormonal knowledge is playing an increasingly crucial role in disease prevention, diagnosis, and therapy, and so, indirectly, in the prolongation and improvement of human life.

A GIANT STEP FORWARD

The development of the technique called radioimmunoassay in the late 1960s provided researchers with an invaluable tool. For the first time, minute quantities in the blood could be accurately identified and measured. Radioactive substances are relatively easy to keep track of. Radioimmunoassay involves a series of procedures in which radioactive, or radiolabeled, substances interact with unknown quantities such as hormones. By monitoring the results, scientists can determine the exact concentration of any substance.

Using this new technique, scientists can now measure nearly every hormone in the blood. They can not only prove the existence of a hormone but also determine its normal levels and the timing of its secretions. Although additional tests are now available to clinicians, radioimmunoassays continue to be extremely important in the calculation of hormonal levels.

GENETIC ADVANCES

As we have seen, replacement, or supplemental, hormonal therapy has an increasingly important place in medicine, such as in the use of insulin to counteract diabetic symptoms, the use of

A scientist prepares a polymerase-chain-reaction machine for a series of gene-amplification cycles. This mechanism allows scientists to amplify a specific DNA sequence millions of times.

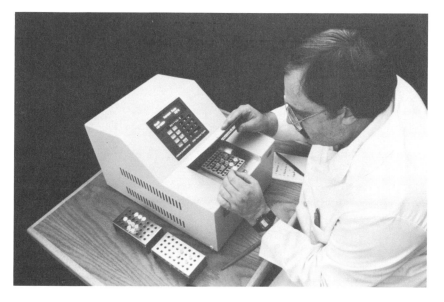

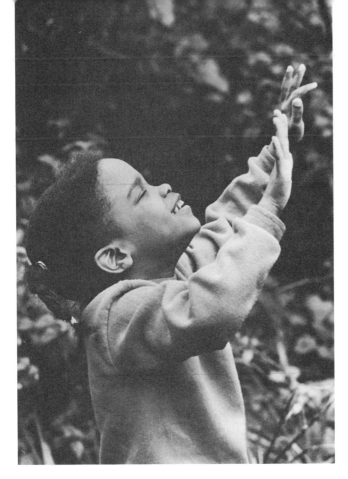

Today's children may someday benefit greatly from scientific advances that can result from a thorough understanding of the endocrine system.

growth hormone as a correction of growth disorders, and the use of estrogen to alter the reproductive cycle in women. But scientists are just beginning to explore the vast therapeutic potential of hormones. Until recently, the lack of available hormones for study severely limited research. In some cases, animals provided reasonable supplies. For example, insulin could be extracted from the pancreas of cows or pigs. For most other hormones, though, sufficient quantities were extremely difficult to obtain. Even if they were found to be highly beneficial, treatments with these hormones were prohibitively expensive.

Two recent breakthroughs offer the promise of unlimited, pure, reasonably priced, readily accessible quantities of all known hormones: *recombinant DNA technology and polymerase chain reaction.* Recombinant DNA technology experts are currently involved in what is called "genetic engineering." They begin by going into the nucleus of a cell. Here, they locate the DNA (deoxyribonucleic acid), genetic material that controls all cell reproduction. Then they identify the exact portion that is in charge of the function or product they wish to duplicate.

Although scientists have just begun to tap this field, they have already made impressive inroads in interpreting DNA. With this new technology, they are able to remove a specific portion of DNA and implant, or recombine, it in the DNA of a rapidly growing culture. Thus, for example, the genetic code for the production of thymosin could be implanted in a rapidly growing yeast cell. As the yeast cell reproduced, so would the quantity of thymosin. After sufficient cycles, the thymosin could be readily separated, purified, and ready for use. This reproduction would supply scientists with unlimited hormonal materials upon which to experiment.

Polymerase chain reaction is a new technology just released by Cetus Laboratories in Emeryville, California, in 1988. This takes recombinant DNA technology one step further; it speeds up the entire process. Using this technology, a billion copies of a particular DNA product can be produced in less than three hours. This is expected to play a crucial role in medical research in the coming decades.

SOME THOUGHTS TO PONDER

As researchers gradually unveil the mysteries of the endocrine system, they are gaining more and more knowledge of how the body functions, and so too, a greater degree of control over how long, and how comfortably, people can live. Millions of people are already benefiting from scientific advances in our knowledge of glands and hormones, and the future shows great promise. In fact, some researchers are beginning to sound much like Professor Brown-Séquard. They speculate that through our grasp of the endocrine system, we will be able to extend our youth, increase our lifespan, change our personality, eliminate disease, and correct many genetic flaws.

In the near future, advances in the field of endocrinology will offer unprecedented opportunities to change and control lives. These discoveries will raise important questions. How long do people want to live? How tall is normal? Should sexuality be controlled? Should differences in personality be subject to hormonal treatments? And most important, who should make these decisions?

Now is the time to ponder the significance of what scientists have uncovered and to consider what their discoveries may lead to in the future.

•   •   •   •

APPENDIX:
FOR MORE INFORMATION

The following is a list of organizations that can provide further information on the endocrine system and the disorders related to dysfunction of endocrine glands.

GENERAL

Canadian Society of Endocrinology
  and Metabolism
Montreal General Hospital
Room 7823-2H
1650 Cedar Avenue
Montreal, Quebec H3G 1A4
Canada
(514) 934-8017

Endocrine Society
9650 Rockville Pike
Bethesda, MD 20814
(301) 571-1802

International Society of
  Endocrinology
Department of Chemical
  Endocrinology
St. Bartholomew's Hospital
51–53 Bartholomew Close
London EC1A 7BEUK
England   01-606-4012

International Stress and Tension
  Control Association
c/o Dr. F. J. McGuigan
Institute of Stress Management
U.S. International University
10455 Pomerado Road
San Diego, CA 92131
(619) 693-4669

Lawson-Wilkins Pediatric
  Endocrine Society
Department of Endocrinology
Children's National Medical Center
111 Michigan Avenue, NW
Washington, DC 20010
(202) 745-2121

National Health Information Center
Office of Disease Prevention and
  Health Promotion
P.O. Box 1133
Washington, DC 20013
(301) 565-4167
(800) 336-4797

National Women's Health Network
224 7th Street, SE
Washington, DC 20003
(202) 543-9222

DIABETES AND HYPOGLYCEMIA

Adrenal Metabolic Research Society
  of the Hypoglycemia Foundation
153 Pawling Avenue
Troy, NY 12180
(418) 272-7154

American Diabetes Association
1660 Duke Street
Alexandria, VA 22314

Hot Line (800) ADA-DISC
(703) 549-1500

Canadian Diabetes Association
78 Bond Street
Toronto, Ontario M5B 2J8
Canada
(416) 362-4440

Juvenile Diabetes Foundation
International
432 Park Avenue South
New York, NY 10016
Hot Line (800) 223-1138
(212) 889-7575

GROWTH HORMONE
DYSFUNCTION AND DWARFISM

Human Growth Foundation
P.O. Box 3090
Falls Church, VA 22043
(703) 883-1773

Little People's Research Fund, Inc.
St. Joseph Hospital
80 Sister Pierre Drive
Towson, MD 21204
(301) 494-0055

PREMENSTRUAL SYNDROME

Premenstrual Syndrome Action
P.O. Box 16292
Irvine, CA 92713
(714) 854-4407

Premenstrual Syndrome Hot Line
(800) 327-8456
(800) 432-2882 in Florida
(Operates 24 hours a day, 7 days a
week providing information on
diagnosis and treatment and
where to receive help locally.)

THYROID

American Thyroid Association
Endocrine-Metabolic Service
Walter Reed Army Medical Center
Washington, DC 20307-500
(202) 576-0747

Thyroid Foundation of America
ACC 730S
Massachusetts General Hospital
Boston, MA 02114
(617) 726-8500

STATE LISTINGS

The following is a list of endocrinology departments or divisions at medical colleges in the United States that are accredited by the Association of American Medical Colleges.

ALABAMA

Division of Endocrinology and
Metabolism
Department of Medicine
University of Alabama at
Birmingham
DB 414
University Station
Birmingham, AL 35294
(205) 934-3410

ARIZONA

Department of Endocrinology
University of Arizona College of
Medicine

Arizona Health Sciences Center
501 N. Campbell Avenue
Tucson, AZ 85724
(602) 626-0111

ARKANSAS

Department of Endocrinology
University of Arkansas College of
Medicine
4301 W. Markham Street, Slot 587
Little Rock, AR 72205
(501) 661-5130

CALIFORNIA

Diabetes and Metabolism Clinic
Stanford University Medical Center

Stanford, CA 94305
(415) 723-6054

Division of Endocrinology
University of California, Los
   Angeles
UCLA School of Medicine
Los Angeles, CA 90024
(213) 825-5366

COLORADO

Department of Endocrinology
University of Colorado School of
   Medicine
4200 E. Ninth Avenue
Denver, CO 80262
(303) 399-1211

CONNECTICUT

Department of Endocrinology
Yale University School of Medicine
333 Cedar Street
New Haven, CT 06510
(203) 785-4181

DISTRICT OF COLUMBIA

Department of Endocrinology
Georgetown University School of
   Medicine
3900 Reservoir Road, NW
Washington, DC 20007
(202) 625-8728

Endocrinology Division
George Washington University
Medical Center
2150 Pennsylvania Avenue, NW
Washington, DC 20037
(202) 676-3695

FLORIDA

Department of Endocrinology
University of Florida College of
   Medicine
Box J-215
J. Hillis Miller Health Center
Gainesville, FL 32610
(904) 392-2616

GEORGIA

Department of Endocrinology
Emory University School of
   Medicine
Atlanta, GA 30322
(404) 588-3645

ILLINOIS

Center for Endocrinology,
   Metabolism & Nutrition
Northwestern University Medical
   School
303 E. Chicago Avenue
Chicago, IL 60611
(312) 908-8023

INDIANA

Endocrinology & Metabolism
   Section
Department of Medicine
Indiana University Medical Center
Emerson Hall 421
545 Barnhill Drive
Indianapolis, IN 46223
(317) 264-8554

IOWA

Department of Endocrinology
University of Iowa College of
   Medicine
100 College of Medicine
   Administration Building
Iowa City, IA 52242
(319) 353-4843

KANSAS

Division of Metabolism,
   Endocrinology, & Genetics
University of Kansas Medical
   Center
39th & Rainbow Boulevard
Kansas City, KS 66103
(913) 588-6043

KENTUCKY

Department of Endocrinology
University of Kentucky College of
   Medicine

800 Rose Street
Lexington, KY 40536
(606) 233-5000

LOUISIANA

Department of Endocrinology
Tulane University School of
  Medicine
1430 Tulane Avenue
New Orleans, LA 70112
(504) 588-5441

MARYLAND

Department of Endocrinology
Johns Hopkins University School of
  Medicine
720 Rutland Avenue
Baltimore, MD 21205
(301) 955-5000

Department of Endocrinology
University of Maryland School of
  Medicine
655 W. Baltimore Street
Baltimore, MD 21201
(301) 528-6219

MASSACHUSETTS

Department of Endocrinology
Harvard Medical School
221 Longwood Avenue
Boston, MA 02115
(617) 732-5661

MICHIGAN

Department of Endocrinology
University of Michigan Medical
  Center
3920 A. Alfred Taubman Health
  Care Center
Ann Arbor, MI 48109
(313) 577-5036

MINNESOTA

Division of Endocrinology
Department of Medicine
University of Minnesota Medical
  School
Minneapolis, MN 55455
(612) 624-5150

MISSISSIPPI

Department of Endocrinology
University of Mississippi Medical
  Center
2500 N. State Street
Jackson, MS 39216
(601) 984-5525

MISSOURI

Department of Endocrinology
Washington University School of
  Medicine
660 S. Euclid Avenue
St. Louis, MO 63110
(314) 362-7617

NEBRASKA

Department of Endocrinology
University of Nebraska College of
  Medicine
42nd Street and Dewey Avenue
Omaha, NE 68105
(402) 559-7229

NEW HAMPSHIRE

Department of Endocrinology
Dartmouth Medical School
Hanover, NH 03756
(603) 646-7505

NEW JERSEY

Department of Endocrinology
University of Medicine and
  Dentistry of New Jersey
Robert Wood Johnson Medical
  School
UMDNJ Medical Education
  Building
New Brunswick, NJ 08903
(201) 456-4300

NEW MEXICO

Division of Endocrinology
Department of Medicine
University of New Mexico School of
  Medicine
Albuquerque, NM 87131
(505) 277-4656

NEW YORK

Department of Endocrinology
Cornell University Medical College
1300 York Avenue
New York, NY 10021
(212) 472-4896

Department of Endocrinology
New York University School of
  Medicine
550 First Avenue
New York, NY 10016
(212) 340-7300

Department of Endocrinology
SUNY Health Science Center at
  Syracuse
College of Medicine
Syracuse, NY 13210
(315) 473-5726

Department of Endocrinology
University of Rochester Medical
  Center
601 Elmwood Avenue
Rochester, NY 14642
(716) 275-2896

NORTH CAROLINA

Department of Endocrinology
Duke University Medical Center
Durham, NC 27710
(919) 684-2498

Department of Endocrinology
University of North Carolina at
  Chapel Hill
School of Medicine
Chapel Hill, NC 27514
(919) 966-3336

NORTH DAKOTA

Department of Endocrinology
University of North Dakota
School of Medicine
UND Medical Education Center
Fargo, ND 58102
(701) 293-4133

OHIO

Department of Endocrinology
Ohio State University Hospitals

N-1111 Doan Hall
410 W. 10th Avenue
Columbus, OH 43210
(614) 421-8730

OKLAHOMA

Department of Endocrinology
Oklahoma Memorial Hospital
P.O. Box 26307
Oklahoma City, OK 73190
(405) 271-5896

OREGON

Department of Endocrinology
Oregon Health Sciences University
  School of Medicine
3181 S.W. Sam Jackson Park Road
Portland, OR 97201
(503) 225-8311

PENNSYLVANIA

Department of Endocrinology
Hospital of the University of
  Pennsylvania
3400 Spruce Street
Philadelphia, PA 19104
(215) 662-3790

Department of Endocrinology
Temple University School of
  Medicine
3400 N. Broad Street
Philadelphia, PA 19140
(215) 221-4046

SOUTH CAROLINA

Department of Endocrinology
Medical University of South
  Carolina
171 Ashley Avenue
Charleston, SC 29425
(803) 792-2528

SOUTH DAKOTA

Department of Endocrinology
University of South Dakota School
  of Medicine
2501 W. 22nd Street
Sioux Falls, SD 57105
(605) 339-6790

TENNESSEE

Department of Endocrinology
Vanderbilt University Medical
    Center
1161 21st Avenue, South
Nashville, TN 37232
(615) 322-4871

TEXAS

Department of Endocrinology
Baylor College of Medicine
One Baylor Plaza
Houston, TX 77225
(713) 792-5508

Department of Endocrinology
University of Texas Health Science
    Center at Dallas
5323 Harry Hines Boulevard
Dallas, TX 75235
(214) 688-3111

UTAH

Department of Endocrinology
University of Utah School of
    Medicine
50 N. Medical Drive
Salt Lake City, UT 84132
(801) 581-7761

VERMONT

Department of Endocrinology
University of Vermont College of
    Medicine
E109 Given Building

Burlington, VT 05405
(802) 656-2530

VIRGINIA

Department of Endocrinology
University of Virginia School of
    Medicine
Box 395, Medical Center
Charlottesville, VA 22908
(804) 924-2656

WASHINGTON

Department of Endocrinology
University of Washington School of
    Medicine
RG-20
Seattle, WA 98195
(206) 543-3293

WEST VIRGINIA

Department of Endocrinology
Marshall University School of
    Medicine
Huntington, WV 25701
(304) 526-0561

WISCONSIN

Department of Endocrinology
University of Wisconsin Medical
    School
1300 University Avenue
Madison, WI 53706
(608) 263-4900

FURTHER READING

GENERAL

Krieger, Dorothy T. *Endocrine Rhythms*. New York: Raven Press, 1979.

Kutsky, Roman J. *Handbook of Vitamins, Minerals, and Hormones.* New York: Van Nostrand Reinhold, 1981

Memmier, Ruth Lundeen, M.D., and Dena Lin Wood. *Structure and Function of the Human Body*. Philadelphia: Lippincott, 1987.

Packard, Mary, and Dora Leder. *From Head to Toes: How Your Body Works*. New York: Simon & Schuster, 1985.

Powis, Raymond L. *The Human Body and Why It Works*. Englewood Cliffs, NJ: Prentice-Hall, 1985.

Tortora, Gerald J. *Principles of Human Anatomy*. New York: Harper & Row, 1986.

PITUITARY GLAND

Ablom, Joan. *Little People in America: The Social Dimensions of Dwarfism*. New York: Praeger, 1984.

Bhatnagar, Ajay S., ed *The Anterior Pituitary Gland*. New York: Raven Press, 1983.

Robbins, R. J., and Schlomo Melmed, eds. *Acromegaly: A Century of Scientific and Clinical Progress*. New York: Plenum, 1987.

THYROID AND PARATHYROID

Hamburger, Joel I. *Your Thyroid Gland: Fact & Fiction*. 2nd ed. Springfield, IL: Thomas, 1975.

Hare, John W., et al. *Signs and Symptoms in Endocrine and Metabolic Disorders*. Philadelphia: Lippincott, 1986.

McMurray, W. C. *Essentials of Human Metabolism: The Relationship of Biochemistry to Human Physiology and Disease*. 2nd ed. New York: Harper & Row, 1983.

Wood, Lawrence, M.D. *Your Thyroid: A Home Reference*. New York: Ballantine, 1987.

ADRENAL GLANDS

Asteria, Mary F. *The Physiology of Stress: With Special Reference to the Neuroendocrine System.* New York: Human Science Press, 1984.

Bedford, Stewart. *Tiger Juice: A Book About Stress for Kids.* Chico, CA: A & S Press, 1981.

Cotman, Carl W., et al. *The Neuro-Immune-Endocrine Connection.* New York: Raven Press, 1987.

James, Vivian H., ed. *The Adrenal Gland.* New York: Raven Press, 1979.

PANCREAS

Ahmed, Paul I., and N. Ahmed, eds. *Coping with Juvenile Diabetes.* Springfield, IL: Thomas, 1985.

American Diabetes Association. *Diabetes in the Family.* New York: Prentice-Hall, 1987.

Bloom, A. *Diabetes Explained.* Boston: MTP Press, 1982.

Born, Dorothy. *Diabetes in the Family.* Englewood Cliffs, NJ: Prentice-Hall, 1982.

Budd, Martin L. *Low Blood Sugar: The Twentieth Century Epidemic.* New York: Sterling, 1983.

Colwell, A. R., Jr. *Understanding Your Diabetes.* Springfield, IL: Thomas, 1978.

Duncan, Theodore G. *The Diabetes Fact Book.* New York: Scribners, 1982.

Fredericks, Carlton, and Herman Goodman. *Low Blood Sugar & You.* New York: Putnam, 1969.

Groth, C. G. *Pancreatic Transplantation.* Philadelphia: Saunders, 1988.

OVARIES AND TESTES

Beard, Mary, and Lindsay Curtis. *Menopause and the Years Ahead.* Tucson, AZ: Fisher Books, 1988.

Bell, Ruth. *Changing Bodies, Changing Lives: A Book for Teens on Sex & Relationships.* New York: Random House, 1988.

Burnett, Raymond. *Menopause: All Your Questions Answered.* Chicago: Contemporary Books, 1987.

Calderone, Mary S., and Eric W. Johnson. *The Family Book About Sexuality*. New York: Harper & Row, 1989.

Campbell, Ann, ed. *The Opposite Sex: The Complete Illustrated Guide to Differences Between the Sexes*. New York: Harper & Row, 1989.

Gosden, R. C. *Biology of Menopause: The Causes and Consequences of Ovarian Ageing*. New York: Academic Press, 1985.

Jovanovic, Lois, M.D., and Genell J. Subak-Sharpe. *Hormones: The Woman's Answerbook*. New York: Fawcett Columbine, 1987.

Marshall, Eliot. "The Drug of Champions." *Science* 242 (October 14, 1988): 183–4.

Marzollo, Jean. *Getting Your Period: A Book About Menstruation*. Illustrated by Kent Williams. New York: Dial, 1989.

Osofsky, Howard J. *The Pregnant Teenager: A Medical, Educational, & Social Analysis*. Springfield, IL: Thomas, 1972.

Taylor, Dena. *Red Flower: Rethinking Menstruation*. Freedom, CA: Crossing Press, 1988.

THYMUS AND PINEAL GLAND

Biggar, W. D., et al. *Thymus Involvement in Immunity and Disease*. New York: Irvington, 1973.

Dwyer, John M., M.D. *The Body at War: The Miracle of the Immune System*. New York: New American Library, 1989.

Fellman, Bruce. "A Clockwork Gland." *Science 85* (May 1985): 77–81.

PICTURE CREDITS

Courtesy Armed Forces Institute of Pathology: pp. 36, 48, 58, 64; E. S. Beckwith/Taurus Photos: p. 15; Catus Corporation: p. 93; Center for Disease Control, Atlanta: p. 87; Laimute E. Druskis/Taurus Photos: pp. 39, 73, 88; Thomas Jefferson University Photo, Thaddeus Govan: p. 89; Library of Congress: pp. 33, 45, 47, 50, 59; Menschenfreund/Taurus Photos: p. 56; Phiz Mezey/Taurus Photos: pp. 74, 94; National Institutes of Health: p. 92; National Library of Medicine: pp. 17, 18, 20; Otis Historical Archives, National Museum of Health and Medicine AFIP: p. 44; Alfred Owczarak/Taurus Photos: p. 91; Reuters/Bettmann: p. 77; Martin M. Rotker/Taurus Photos: pp. 43, 61, 78; Taurus Photos: pp. 67, 69; UPI/Bettmann: pp. 13, 25, 31, 35, 76; Shirley Zeiberg/Taurus Photos: p. 65; original illustrations by Nisa Rauschenberg: pp. 14, 21, 23, 27, 28, 30, 41, 53, 63, 71, 83, 85

GLOSSARY

adrenal cortex the outer portion of the adrenal glands; produces aldosterone, cortisol, and other hormones that serve metabolic functions

adrenaline epinephrine; a hormone that is produced in the adrenal medulla and works in conjunction with noradrenaline; causes blood vessel constriction, increased heart and metabolic rates, and other actions that provide the body with extra energy in emergency situations

adrenal medulla the inner portion of the adrenal glands; produces adrenaline and noradrenaline, hormones that help the body combat stress

AIDS acquired immune deficiency syndrome; an acquired defect in the immune system, caused by the virus HIV and spread by blood or sexual contact; leaves people vulnerable to certain, often fatal, infections and cancers

anabolic steroid any of a group of usually synthetic hormones that increases metabolism

androgens sex hormones, the most common of which is testosterone, produced in the testes of males and the adrenal glands of both men and women

B lymphocytes B cells; white blood cells that produce antibodies and work in conjunction with T cells

diabetes insipidus a rare disease caused by insufficient amounts of antidiuretic hormone; characterized by polydipsia and polyuria

diabetes mellitus a hereditary endocrine disorder classified into two types: type I (juvenile-onset) is usually caused by deficient insulin production; type II (adult-onset) is caused by the body's inability to use insulin; both types are characterized by excessive amounts of sugar in the blood and urine, severe thirst, hunger, and weight loss

dwarfism the condition of being abnormally small; among its many causes are kidney insufficiency, skeletal disease, and the insufficient release of growth hormone during childhood

endocrine system the system of glands located throughout the body that produces hormones and secretes them directly into the bloodstream; plays a key role in growth, reproduction, metabolism, and immune system actions

gland a bodily structure that secretes a substance, especially one it has extracted from the blood and altered for subsequent secretion

goiter an enlargement of the thyroid gland, often caused by iodine deficiency and resulting in a swelling of the front part of the neck

growth hormone GH; somatotropin; a hormone produced in the anterior pituitary that regulates and stimulates growth until maturity

hormone a product of the endocrine glands that circulates freely throughout the bloodstream, controlling and regulating other glands and organs by chemical stimulation

hyperglycemia abnormally increased glucose content in the blood; an early symptom of diabetes mellitus

hypoglycemia abnormally diminished concentration of glucose in the blood; caused by excessive insulin levels, either organically produced or medically administered; symptoms include fatigue, anxiety, blurred vision, and headaches

hypothalamus the section of the brain that controls the pituitary gland; regulates survival processes, such as reproduction, nourishment, and self-defense, by initiating the appropriate physical response through nerve impulses and chemical messengers

insulin a hormone secreted by the pancreas that regulates the metabolism of carbohydrates and the maintenance of blood sugar levels

islet of Langerhans any of a cluster of nearly a million cells located in the pancreas; secretes hormones such as insulin and glucagon

melatonin a hormone produced in the pineal gland and secreted only in the absence of light; thought to influence sexual activity, concentration ability, the need for sleep, and the desire for carbohydrates

menopause cessation of menstruation by natural causes; usually occurs between the ages of 45 and 50

menstruation the cyclic shedding of the uterine lining that occurs in the absence of pregnancy during the reproductive period (puberty through menopause) of the female

neuron nerve cell; the basic component of the nervous system; operates by carrying electrical messages throughout the body with great speed and efficiency

noradrenalin norepinephrine; a hormone that is produced in the adrenal medulla and works in conjunction with adrenalin; causes increased blood pressure and breathing rate, as well as other reactions that enable the body to respond to stress

ovaries the pair of female reproductive glands located in the lower abdomen; produce eggs and the hormones estrogen and progesterone

ovulation release of an egg cell, or ovum, from the ovaries into the oviduct; the result of a chain reaction that begins with a chemical message from the endocrine system

pancreas the body's second-largest gland, it is also an organ; produces insulin and glucagon, the hormones primarily responsible for balancing the body's blood sugar level

parathyroid gland four small organs, situated at the back of the thyroid, that secrete parathyroid hormone and are chiefly concerned with the metabolism of calcium and phosphorous

pituitary gland "the master gland"; a small gland located in the brain, attached to the hypothalamus, and composed of two sections: the anterior lobe and posterior lobe; controls the thyroid, adrenal, and sex glands

PMS premenstrual syndrome; a physical and emotional condition caused by the surge and fall of hormonal levels during the course of the menstrual cycle; common symptoms include soreness, bloating, tension, and irritability

puberty the period of rapid growth during which secondary sex characteristics develop and the capability of sexual reproduction is attained; its onset, which is stimulated by a sudden increase in the production of sex hormones, generally occurs in females between the ages of 8 and 14 and in males in their early teens

SAD seasonal affective disorder; a form of depression afflicting some people during the long, dark winter months; its intensity correlates to the increase in melatonin production brought on by diminished light and is alleviated largely by light-treatment therapy

testes testicles; the pair of male sex organs located in the scrotum; produce sperm and testosterone

testosterone hormone produced in the testes of males and the adrenal glands of both males and females; responsible for the development of male secondary sex characteristics

thymus glandular structure in the chest where T cells mature; an essential part of the immune system

thyroid a glandular structure located at the base of the neck; regulates growth and many of the metabolic processes

INDEX

Marjorie Little, a free-lance science writer and member of the American Medical Writers Association, received her M.S. degree in sociology from the University of Pittsburgh. She is the author of the ImmunoPrimer Series, a six-part tutorial on immunology research written for medical professionals, and the editor of *AIDS: You Can't Catch It Holding Hands*.

Dale C. Garell, M.D., is medical director of California Children Services, Department of Health Services, County of Los Angeles. He is also associate dean for curriculum at the University of Southern California School of Medicine and clinical professor in the Department of Pediatrics & Family Medicine at the University of Southern California School of Medicine. From 1963 to 1974, he was medical director of the Division of Adolescent Medicine at Children's Hospital in Los Angeles. Dr. Garell has served as president of the Society for Adolescent Medicine, chairman of the youth committee of the American Academy of Pediatrics, and as a forum member of the White House Conference on Children (1970) and White House Conference on Youth (1971). He has also been a member of the editorial board of the *American Journal of Diseases of Children*.

C. Everett Koop, M.D., Sc.D., is former Surgeon General, Deputy Assistant Secretary for Health, and Director of the Office of International Health of the U.S. Public Health Service. A pediatric surgeon with an international reputation, he was previously surgeon-in-chief of Children's Hospital of Philadelphia and professor of pediatric surgery and pediatrics at the University of Pennsylvania. Dr. Koop is the author of more than 175 articles and books on the practice of medicine. He has served as surgery editor of the *Journal of Clinical Pediatrics* and editor-in-chief of the *Journal of Pediatric Surgery*, Dr. Koop has received nine honorary degrees and numerous other awards, including the Denis Brown Gold Medal of the British Association of Paediatric Surgeons, the William E. Ladd Gold Medal of the American Academy of Pediatrics, and the Copernicus Medal of the Surgical Society of Poland. He is a Chevalier of the French Legion of Honor and a member of the Royal College of Surgeons, London.